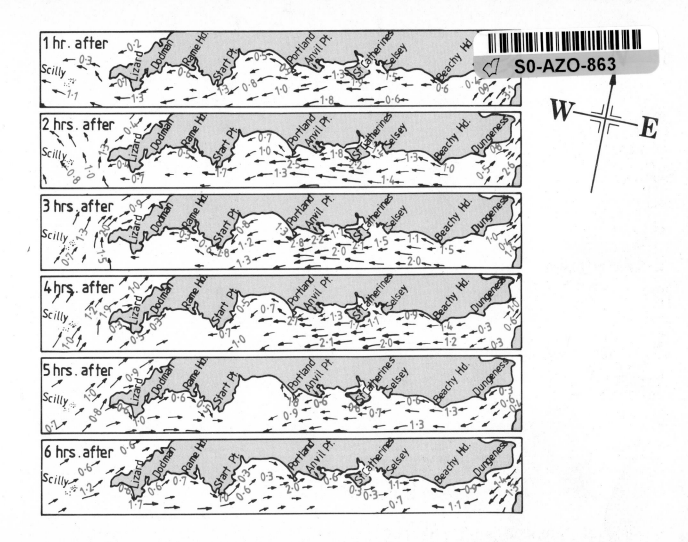

The Shell Pilot to the English Channel

The Shell Pilot to the English Channel

1. Harbours on the South Coast of England

Ramsgate to the Scillies

Captain J. O. Coote, Royal Navy

with plans by James Petter

based on earlier editions by

K. Adlard Coles

A Shell Guide

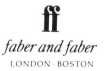

faber and faber
LONDON · BOSTON

First published as *Sailing on the South Coast* in 1937
Reissued 1939
by Faber and Faber Limited
3 Queen Square London WC1N 3AU
Second edition, with new title, 1950
Pocket Pilot for the South Coast
Third edition 1962
Fourth edition, wholly revised, 1968
Reprinted, with new title, 1971
The Shell Pilot to the South Coast Harbours
Interim edition, with correction pages, 1973
Fifth edition, wholly revised, 1977
Sixth edition, wholly revised, 1982
Interim edition, with correction pages and new title, 1985
Seventh edition, wholly revised, 1987
The Shell Pilot to the English Channel
1. Harbours on the South Coast of England: Ramsgate to the Scillies
Reprinted with list of errata, 1989
Eighth edition, wholly revised, 1990
Photoset by Wilmaset, Birkenhead, Wirral
Printed in Great Britain by Clays Ltd, St Ives plc

A CIP record for this book is available from the British Library

ISBN 0-571-14430-6

To
DAVID CURLING

Contents

*Harbours which are not accessible at all states of weather or tide.
See at the start of each relevant section for precautions to be observed.

Preface

This is the eighth edition of the book which originally appeared in 1937 as *Sailing on the South Coast* by the redoubtable K. Adlard Coles. It is a complete revision of *The Shell Pilot to the English Channel – Harbours on the South Coast of England* which first came out in 1985 as a companion volume to the then new work *Harbours in Northern France and the Channel Islands*. Both are a tribute to Shell's enduring sponsorship and to Adlard's pioneer work in this field, from which sprang the whole range of today's pilotage books for yachtsmen.

The need for another edition of the South Coast pilotage book has once again been dictated by major changes in many harbours and their approaches. There seems to be no end to the continuing demand for alongside berths for yachts whose owners are prepared to pay for the privilege of driving through holiday traffic to park their cars near by and walk on board, without resorting to using overloaded dinghies. Not only have new marinas appeared in Portsmouth, Bembridge, Brixham and Falmouth, but there has been a growth in the compromise of providing berths alongside pontoons which are securely moored in a quiet corner of the anchorage. Sometimes these are served by water-taxis. Many new marinas are firmly linked to major waterfront property developments, with no long-term provision for visitors' berths. At last there is a viable plan to add a major marina in Cowes protected from gales from any direction. That will be the case when the old Westland Hovercraft factory water frontage is linked to reclaimed land where The Shrape has for a century lured tide-dodging keelboats to an all-standing stop.

It may be bad news in the *Guide Michelin* to remove a rosette, but I am delighted to delete the cautionary asterisk (denoting access limited by weather or tide conditions) from Bembridge, which now has a straight 2m0 channel leading to the dredged eastern end of the harbour and a marina alongside the new premises planned for the Bembridge SC as part of the deal.

One major new marina project forecast in the last edition has not so far come to pass – that in Haslar Creek opposite the submarine base at *HMS Dolphin*. There are signs that the high cost of money and the recession in the property market are having their depressing effect, which may postpone the need for a ninth edition of this book for longer than has been the case in recent years.

This edition has several new bird's-eye shots taken by Sealand Aerial Photography, of Goodwood airport, and introduces two new picture contributors: Roger Lean-Vercoe of Yealmpton and my former Express Newspapers' colleague John Robertson during a brief escape from the Costa del Sol. Most of the new sea-level pictures have been taken by me on a painfully-slow learning curve, sometimes in boats I have chartered but often in the agreeable company of David Curling in his Beneteau 32 *Nephele*.

The popularity of VHF radio-telephones still increases. Most harbour authorities are available to give advice on berthing to those who call when approaching a new port. Channel 37 (the Marina band on 157.850 MHz) is becoming overcrowded, so Channel 80 (161.625 MHz) is increasingly used as an alternative. It will become mandatory from April 1991.

James Petter, of Petersfield, the young engineering draughtsman who turned cartographer for the 1982 edition, has once again done an impeccable job. Nearly all the charts needed amending, while ten of them had to be redrawn from scratch. One new chart has been added to enable yachtsmen to enjoy a trip up the River Exe as far as Topsham.

I am greatly indebted to the Controller of Her Majesty's

Stationery Office, the Hydrographer of the Navy, Imray Laurie Norie & Wilson Ltd and Barnacle Marine Ltd, publishers of Stanfords charts, for complementing my own observations with their reliable source-data. On this occasion the times of High and Low Water Dover for 1991 have been produced to my format by the Proudman Oceanographic Laboratory, Bidston Observatory. They are now supplied as a loose insert, which will be replaced on demand each succeeding year during the lifetime of this edition.

Yachtsmen could also profitably turn to many locally-produced information booklets, such as the *Solent Year Book*, *Chichester Harbour Guide*, the *Sailing and Boating Guide to the Fal Area* and Norm's *Yachtsman's Guide to Scilly*.

The passage of time and each weekly edition of *Notices to Mariners* may throw up the need for further revisions, but every endeavour has been made to ensure this book's accuracy at the time of its going to the printers at Whitsun 1990. In all of this I have been greatly assisted by my wife, Sylvia, who has contrived to deliver order out of the chaos of my study and has in turn acted as researcher, driver, shipmate and progress-chaser during the fieldwork period.

This publication has two companion volumes: Part 2 of *The Shell Pilot to the English Channel* covering harbours in Northern France and the Channel Islands; and *The Shell Guide to Yacht Navigation*, a primer for the amateur navigator who is bewildered by the seemingly irrelevant theory of celestial navigation and the whole array of electronic nav-aids. It is hoped that he will profit by all my mistakes and possibly develop a healthy scepticism towards the infallibility claimed by the manufacturers of push-button position-finders.

Wherever you sail, this book on its own is not enough. Be sure to have a copy of the local by-laws governing any port to be visited. It should always be assumed that Rule 9(b) of the Regulations for Preventing Collisions at Sea applies. It is sometimes known as the Gross Registered Tonnage Law:

A vessel of under 20 metres in length or a sailing vessel shall not impede the passage of a vessel which can safely navigate only within a narrow channel or fairway.

Readers are invited to contribute any corrections, new information or constructive criticism to me at Titty Hill Farm, Iping, Midhurst, W. Sussex GU29 0PL.

John Coote
June 1990

Explanation of Terms, Chart Symbols and Abbreviations

Charts referred to: BA are British Admiralty charts.
Im are those from Imray.
Stan are Stanfords charts.

Times of High Water The average time differences for each harbour applied to the time of HW Dover have been supplied by the Institute of Oceanographic Sciences, or have been estimated where data are not available. To arrive at the time of HW in a harbour, take the time of HW at Dover and add or subtract the difference shown in the introductory notes for each port covered by this book. These constants are only approximate; for greater accuracy, where harbours are a long way from Dover, look up the predicted times of HW for the nearest standard port in Admiralty Tide Tables and then apply the time difference for whichever secondary port you are interested in. Nearly all ports have their own local tide tables, generally available at the harbour office, marinas or local newsagents.

Double High Waters occur at Southampton, in the West Solent ports and are even more evident in Christchurch and Poole. For these harbours the first HW at spring tides is included in the tidal data; in the Solent the second HW occurs about 2 hours later. HW at Neap tides is always later than first HW Springs, but there are long stands of tide, sometimes existing for several hours. Hence the average times of local HW referred to Dover would at best be approximations. However, predictions for each day of the year can be found in ATT.

Charted Depths and Data The charted depths given in this book are shown in metres; they indicate the depth of water *below chart datum* which is reduced to the level of LAT, or the drying heights (figures underlined) above it. Figures are given in the tidal data for each harbour for extra water at MHWS, MLWS, MHWN and MLWN which may be added to the charted depths or interpolated for intermediate states of tide. It will be noted that in many harbours om6 (2 ft) may be added to the charted depths at MLWS and as much as 1m8 (6 ft) at MLWN; these are of great significance when navigating in shallow channels. Also note that tidal levels may be affected by weather conditions. For example, fresh northerly to easterly winds may bring low runs of tide sometimes lowering the levels to the extent of om6 (2 ft).

Heights of conspicuous landmarks other than lighthouses are shown in brackets in metres. Thus 'Chy (99)' indicates a chimney 99 metres above sea-level at its top. The same convention is used to indicate safe clearances under a bridge or overhead cable at MHWS.

Distances at sea are expressed in nautical miles or cables; on land in statute miles and kilometres.

Bearings and Courses Distances are given in nautical miles, cables and metres. Bearings and courses are True, to which Variation must be added and Deviation applied for ship's magnetic compass readings.

Approach The directions assume that the vessel is approaching from seaward, and objects are described on the port or starboard hand of a ship entering the harbour.

Chart Symbols – Lights Lights outside harbours only are shown, except (1) leading lights placed inside, and (2) important buoys used for proceeding up harbour.

Lights are symbolized, the word 'light' or 'Lt' omitted. The characteristic of each light is noted, e.g. F for fixed, Gp Fl or Fl is group flashing, etc., and in the case of other than white lights, the colour, e.g. R, G, etc., followed by elevation in metres (m) and range (M) miles. Bearings are generally expressed to the nearest degree true, and cardinal or half cardinal points are used only to indicate approximate directions. The limits of sectors and arcs of visibility and the alignment of directional lights and leading lights are given as *seen by an observer from seaward* as true compass bearings.

Buoys are symbolized, and the word 'buoy' omitted. Colour and shape are not always described, but symbol conforms to shape of buoy and, where scale allows, to configuration, i.e. solid black for green buoys, outline or patched shading for white or red, chequers and stripes shown as such. The positions of mooring buoys cannot always be shown on the harbour plans, often being precluded by scale, but visitors' moorings are referred to in the text.

Beacons are either symbolized as Bn or shown as small round 'o'. The point where pole crosses base line indicates exact position.

Coloured Area Heavy stipple indicates parts which dry out at LAT. Green indicates water where there is less than 2 metres at LAT and is bounded by dotted line. All depths over 2 metres are left white.

Anchorage Symbol (⚓) is intended to draw attention to proximity of anchorage, and does not necessarily indicate the precise or only spot for letting go. Anchorages are being increasingly occupied by moorings, but are referred to in the text.

Minor posts, withies, dolphins, etc., inside harbours are sometimes precluded by scale.

Abbreviations – Tidal

ATT	Admiralty Tide Tables
HW	High Water
LW	Low Water
LAT	Lowest Astronomical Tide
CD	Chart datum
MHWS	Mean High Water Springs
MHWN	Mean High Water Neaps
MLWS	Mean Low Water Springs
MLWN	Mean Low Water Neaps

Other Abbreviations

Alt	Alternating
B	Black
Bn	Beacon
Bu	Blue
BuW	Blue and White
BW	Black and White
BY	Black and Yellow
Cheq	Chequers
con	conical
dia	diaphone
Dir	Directional
ev	every
F	Fixed
Fl	Flashing
FS	Flagstaff
G	Green
Gp	Group
H	Horizontal
h.	hour(s)
HM	Harbour Master
HO	Harbour Office
IntQ	Interrupted Quick Flashing

Iso	Isophase	
km	kilometres	
kt	knot	
LFl	Long Flashing	
Lt	Light	
Lt Ho	Lighthouse	
LV	Light-vessel	
m	metres	
m.	minutes (time)	
M	Miles (nautical)	
Mag	Magnetic	
Mo	Morse Code Signal	
NB	Notice Board	
Oc	Occulting	
Occas	Occasional	
Or	Orange	
PA	Position approximate	
Q	Quick Flashing	
R	Red	
Ra Refl	Radar Reflector	
Ro Bn	Radio Beacon	
RW	Red and White	
RY	Red and Yellow	
S	Stripes	
SC	Sailing Club	
s.	seconds (time)	
Sph	Spherical	
Tr	Tower	
Vert	Vertical	

vis	visible
VQ	Very Quick Flashing
W	White
Y	Yellow
YC	Yacht Club
∅	Transit
→	Right-hand edge
←	Left-hand edge
Ⓥ	Visitors' berths

VHF Voice Frequencies

Ch	5	160.850 (Weymouth Bay)
	9	156.450 MHz
	10	156.500
	11	156.550
	12	156.600
	13	156.650
	14	156.700
	16	156.800 (Distress and Calling)
	26	157.300 (Start Pt)
	27	157.350 (Land's End)
	28	157.400 (Niton)
	37	157.850 (Marina band)
	62	160.725 (Pendennis)
	67	156.375 (Coastguards)
	70	156.525 (Distress and Safety exclusive)
	74	156.725 (Dover)
	80	161.625 (Alternate Marina band)
	88	162.025 (VHF Lt Ho see p. 16)

Conversions

Cable = 0.1 M	200 yds	182 m
Nautical Mile	1.85 km	1.14 stat. miles
Statute Mile	1.69 km	0.88 M
Fathom	1.83 metres	

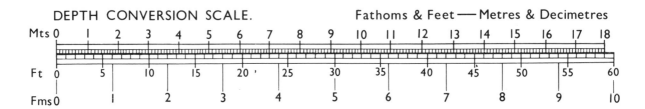

DEPTH CONVERSION SCALE.   Fathoms & Feet ——— Metres & Decimetres

Mts 0 1 2 3 4 5 6 7 8 9 10 11 12 13 14 15 16 17 18

Ft 0   5   10   15   20   25   30   35   40   45   50   55   60

Fms 0   1   2   3   4   5   6   7   8   9   10

Tide Tables

The loose card gives the times and heights of High and Low Water DOVER for 1991. The times of High Water (HW) are shown on green tint throughout. They may be used in conjunction with the South Coast tidal charts inside the front cover and the times and heights given for each harbour in this book.

Times are expressed in four figures as clock time, the necessary adjustment having been made for BST.

Datum of Predictions is also Chart Datum which is 3.67 metres below Ordnance Datum at Newlyn.

Depths and heights are given in metres to one place of decimals.

Copyright. Tidal Predictions published herein have been computed by the Institute of Oceanographic Sciences, Bidston Observatory, Birkenhead, copyright reserved.

The following conversion table is for use with the Tide Tables:

Metres	Feet/inches	Metres	Feet/inches
0.1	0'4"	1.0	3'3"
0.2	0'8"	2.0	6'7"
0.3	1'0"	3.0	9'10"
0.4	1'4"	4.0	13'1"
0.5	1'8"	5.0	16'5"
0.6	2'0"	6.0	19'8"
0.7	2'4"	7.0	23'0"
0.8	2'8"	8.0	26'3"
0.9	2'11"	9.0	29'6"

Radio Wavelength/Frequency Conversion Table (in MF band)

Metres	kHz	Metres	kHz	Metres	kHz
100	3000	250	1200	400	750
125	2400	275	1100	425	700
150	2000	300	1000	450	665
175	1710	325	930	475	630
200	1500	350	855	500	600
225	1340	375	800	525	

BBC Shipping Forecast on Long 1515 metres = 198 kHz

VHF Radio Lighthouses: Channel 88 (162.025 MHz)

For boats with VHF radio able to receive Ch 88 (162.025 MHz) there are some VHF shore transmitters which will give their bearing from seaward to an accuracy of 2 degrees, regardless of the motion or compass heading of the receiving boat. Quadrantal errors and the effect of uninsulated guardrails or wraparound metal construction are also irrelevant.

The operation is simple: on acquiring the signal, which leads off with the Morse call sign, start counting the beats until there is a sudden null. By reference to the tables below the bearing of the VHF lighthouse ashore is thus obtained in degrees (true) from seaward. Its range is governed by line-of-sight propagation, so those shown on the tables below are approximate, depending, *inter alia*, on the height of your own VHF antenna. **Bearings taken at greater ranges are subject to significant errors.** It is possible that further stations may be established at the Casquets, Penlee Pt (Plymouth) and on the Cherbourg Peninsula.

Bearing of Lt Ho from Seaward in Degrees True

	Beats	0	1	2	3	4	5	6	7	8	9
V3 Anvil Point Lt Ho	0	–	–	–	–	–	–	–	247	249	251
Call sign: AL (._ ._..)	10	253	255	257	259	261	263	265	267	269	271
Range: 14M	20	273	275	277	279	281	283	285	287	289	291
Alternate with	30	293	295	297	299	301	303	305	307	309	311
Scratchells Bay (V6)	40	313	315	317	319	321	323	325	327	329	331
	50	333	335	337	339	341	343	345	347	349	351
	60	353	355	357	359	001	003	005	007	–	–
V6 Scratchells Bay	0	–	–	–	–	–	–	–	337	339	341
0.4M Needles Lt 280°	10	343	345	347	349	351	353	355	357	359	001
Call sign: HD (.... _..)	20	003	005	007	009	011	013	015	017	019	021
Range: 30M	30	023	025	027	029	031	033	035	037	039	041
Alternate with	40	043	045	047	049	051	053	055	057	059	061
Anvil Point Lt (V3)	50	063	065	067	069	071	073	075	077	079	081
	60	083	085	087	089	091	093	095	097	–	–

Part One

Passage Data and Principal Headlands

Distances are given in nautical miles.
Courses and bearings in degrees True.

Tidal charts
The English Channel inside front cover.
The Isle of Wight on p. 26.
Around Portland Bill on p. 31.

Tides off other headlands are dealt with in the text.

Customs and Immigration Contact the local Harbour Office or dial 100 and ask for Freephone Customs Yachts before sailing. Complete Form C1328 Part 1, hand it in or deposit in the special mail-box provided for the purpose at all marinas. Check that all have in-date passports.

On return, fly Flag Q until specifically cleared by Customs and the rest of Form C1328 is dealt with. Failure to do so can lead to prosecution, a hefty fine and life membership of an unenviable club – the Customs' Black List. If you want to alert the Customs to your ETA on return, it is necessary to make a linked call by radio telephone, if the local Harbour Office cannot do so for you. Each major port's Customs number is listed, or they may be contacted by areas:

Land's End – Exmouth	0752–669811
Lyme Regis – Weymouth	03057–71189
Poole – Newhaven	0703–229251
Rye – Ramsgate	0304–202441

The Channel Islands count as abroad for these purposes. The Q Flag is not insisted upon on arrival at French ports unless you have something to declare. French authorities like to see the originals (rather than copies) of ship's papers and evidence that no charter business is being originated there.

Coastguard Service Although many CG stations may be manned during emergencies or for exercises, 24-hour watches are now only kept at Marine Rescue Co-ordination Centres (MRCC) and at Maritime Rescue Sub-Centres (MRSC). They all listen on Ch 16. Those along the South Coast may be contacted by telephone direct or through linked calls as follows:

MRCC Dover	0304–210008
MRSC Lee-on-Solent	0705–552100
MRSC Portland	0305–820441
MRSC Brixham	08045–58292
MRCC Falmouth	0326–317575

or call on 999 from ashore.

At some time you may be involved in a rescue. The CG would like to have full particulars of your boat on their files. You can help by picking up a postcard wherever you see the white-on-red disc 'H. M. Coastguard Yacht and Boat Safety Scheme – Issuing Authority', completing it and mailing it to the nearest CG station. On a long passage make contact by radio as you pass through an area.

Weather Forecasts Besides the Shipping Forecasts on BBC 198 kHz (1515 m) and local sources of met. data given after each port in Part Two, there is a new telephone service, MARINE-CALL, which has replaced the short-lived MARINELINE. It is obtained by calling 0898–500, followed by 3 digits for the area required:

456 Selsey – N. Foreland; Le Havre – Calais.
457 Lyme Regis – Selsey; Cherbourg and Channel Islands.
458 Hartland Point – Lyme Regis; Brittany.

It is not cheap (38p peak times, 25p evenings and weekends), but it is updated hourly, on continuous transmission, and distinguishes between coastal waters on opposite sides of the Channel (a weakness of the BBC broadcasts).

Charts Before you buy any others, one or more of the following are desirable for planning purposes:

BA 2675	English Channel
Im C10	English Channel passage chart – western section (Scillies to Owers).
Im C12	English Channel passage chart – eastern section (Portland to North Foreland).
Stan 1	English Channel eastern section (Anvil Point to North Foreland).
Stan 2	English Channel western section (Scillies to Owers).

The shortest navigable distances on the rhumb-line
between safe distances off each headland

N. FORELAND	N. FORELAND													
DUNGENESS	36	DUNGENESS												
BEACHY HEAD	66	30	BEACHY HEAD											
OWERS	101	65	35	OWERS										
ST CATHERINE'S	125	89	59	24	ST CATHERINE'S									
ANVIL POINT	150	114	84	49	25	ANVIL POINT								
PORTLAND BILL	170	134	104	69	45	20	PORTLAND BILL							
BERRY HEAD	210	174	144	109	85	60	40	BERRY HEAD						
START POINT	218	182	152	117	93	68	48	13	START POINT					
BOLT HEAD	224	188	158	123	99	74	54	19	6	BOLT HEAD				
RAME HEAD	242	206	176	141	117	92	72	36	23	17	RAME HEAD			
DODMAN	263	227	197	162	138	113	93	57	45	39	24	DODMAN		
LIZARD	282	246	215	181	156	132	111	75	62	56	44	22	LIZARD	
RUNNEL STONE	300	265	234	200	175	151	130	94	81	75	63	42	19	RUNNEL STONE
BISHOP ROCK	330	294	263	229	204	180	159	123	111	105	93	71	48	32	BISHOP ROCK

The shortest navigable distances on the rhumb-line between harbour entrances or bars

	RAMSGATE	BRIGHTON	CHICHESTER	PORTSMOUTH	COWES	LYMINGTON	POOLE	WEYMOUTH	DARTMOUTH	SALCOMBE	PLYMOUTH	FOWEY	FALMOUTH	PENZANCE
RAMSGATE														
BRIGHTON	78													
CHICHESTER	112	34												
PORTSMOUTH	119	41	7											
COWES	125	47	15	8										
LYMINGTON	132	56	24	17	9									
POOLE	152	74	42	35	27	19								
WEYMOUTH	173	97	64	57	49	40	27							
DARTMOUTH	212	135	107	100	92	84	70	52						
SALCOMBE	220	144	117	110	103	95	81	64	14					
PLYMOUTH	241	165	135	132	123	115	98	82	35	17				
FOWEY	255	178	152	144	139	129	116	96	48	36	20			
FALMOUTH	271	194	168	160	152	143	130	113	63	50	38	20		
PENZANCE	295	219	190	183	176	168	155	135	88	74	64	48	32	
SCILLY	322	246	218	211	204	195	183	163	116	102	92	76	60	37

Principal Headlands

Charts: BA 1828; Im C8; Stan 9

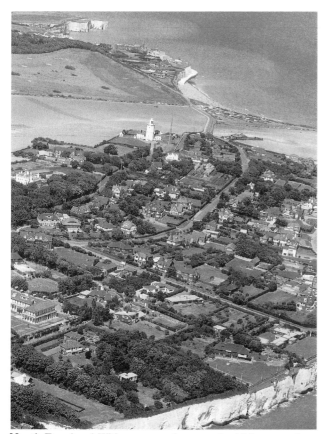

North Foreland Conspicuous 26m white 8-sided light tower (Fl (5) WR 20s. 57m 21M) on bold, nearly perpendicular chalk cliffs. At position 3.2 miles 141° from headland: north-going stream −0120 Dover; south-going stream +0440 Dover. Springs 2¾ knots.

South Foreland Bold irregular chalk cliff over 90m high. Two lighthouses on the summit, both now disused. The Western Lt. 21m white square castellated tower. Tidal streams between South Foreland and Deal: north-going about −0145 Dover: south-going about +0415 Dover, spring rate 2¼ knots.

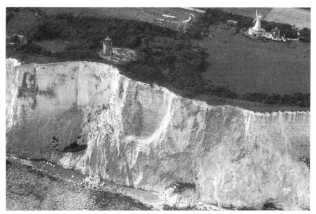

North Foreland *White octagonal tower 26m high, 57 m above sea-level*

South Foreland *White square castellated tower 21m high, 114m above sea-level. Its light has been extinguished*

23

Dungeness A low promontory with steep beach at its south-east end. Prominent lighthouse (Fl W 10s. 40m 27M. Horn (3) 60s.) black round tower, white bands. 40m elevation. Old lighthouse and nuclear power station adjacent to west. Anchorage in roads on either side of Dungeness according to direction of wind. At position 2.4M 140° from Dungeness High lighthouse the east stream begins −0200 Dover. West stream +0430 Dover. Spring rate of about 2 knots.

Beachy Head This is a very prominent chalk headland. About a mile west of the head is a disused lighthouse, but the operative lighthouse (Fl (2) W 20s. 31m 25M Horn 30s.) is situated off the rocks below Beachy Head which extend seaward; to the south-east of Beachy Head there are the rocks known as the Head Ledge extending some ½ mile from the cliffs. The lighthouse tower has a broad red band and an elevation of 43m. Seven miles east of Beachy Head are the Royal Sovereign shoals with 3m8 least water over which there are overfalls. They are marked on the southward side by a prominent light tower (Fl 20s. 28m 28M. dia (2) 30s.)

Beachy Head should be given a berth of 2 miles in heavy weather as there are overfalls and rough water to the southward of it. Two miles south of the lighthouse the streams are east −0520 Dover, spring rate 2.6 knots; west +0015 Dover, spring rate 2 knots.

Selsey Bill and the Owers Selsey Bill is a low sharp point which is difficult to locate if the visibility is poor. There is a conspicuous hotel on the west side of the point. Southward of the Bill there are groups of rocks and ledges between which lie

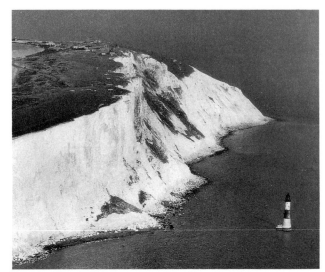

Beachy Head *White tower with red band and lantern 43m high, seen from the south-west*

Looe channel and 7 miles south-east of Selsey Bill the Owers Lanby (Fl (3) W 20s. 12m 22M Horn (3) 60s.) is moored. By keeping south of the light buoy danger is avoided, but in clear weather and moderate winds the Looe channel, which is marked by buoys, affords a short cut, with the aid of a large-scale chart. Tidal streams in the Looe channel: east +0445 Dover; west −0120 Dover. Rate at springs 2.6 knots but faster between the Malt Owers and the Boulder bank. There are local variations in the directions of the streams. Three miles south of the Owers light buoy the tidal streams are west-south-west −0050 Dover; east-north-east +0540 Dover; 2½ to 3 knots at springs.

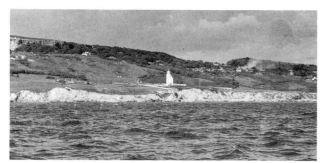

St Catherine's Point *White octagonal castellated tower 26m above sea-level. Not very conspicious by day*

St Catherine's Point   This point is at the southern extremity of the Isle of Wight and lies comparatively low at the foot of the hill which forms the highest part of the island. The lighthouse is a 26m octagonal castellated tower standing at the back of the cliffs; its light is FlW 5s. 41m 30M. It has a 17m R sector (099°–116°) to stop you hitting Rocken End (only 2 cables west of the Point!).

There is a tide race off St Catherine's owing to the uneven bottom in strong streams. This can be very rough under wind against tide conditions and should be avoided; it is dangerous in bad weather. The turbulence of the race varies according to wind, tide and swell and is sometimes rougher or calmer than may be anticipated from the conditions. There are also overfalls to the eastward of St Catherine's off Dunnose and a number of isolated tide rips which locally may be almost as rough as St Catherine's race. Tidal streams between St Catherine's Point and Dunnose: east +0515 Dover; west −0015 Dover; maximum spring rate about 5 knots, weaker seaward.

The Needles Rocks   The sharp white Needles rocks with the lighthouse (Oc (2) WRG 20s. 24m 17M. Horn (2) 30s.) at their seaward end are notable landmarks, but they are by no means conspicuous from a distance in hazy weather. From the west or south-west it is the high white cliffs above Scratchell's Bay just south-east of the Needles which will first be seen, and the high down 3 miles east on which stands Tennyson's Cross. Tidal stream charts should be referred to in the approaches to the Solent from the west, as the streams are strong. The main flood stream from Durlston Head runs east-north-east towards the Needles, where the stream divides. The stronger flood stream runs north-east into the Needles Channel while farther south the stream runs east to south-east off the Isle of Wight coast. Conversely on the ebb the local streams join west of the Needles and set west-south-west towards Durlston Head.

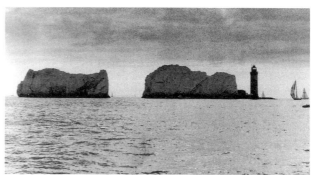

The Needles *33m white tower with red band seen from the north-west. White rocks and cliffs visible by day at extreme range*

TIDAL STREAMS AROUND THE ISLE OF WIGHT

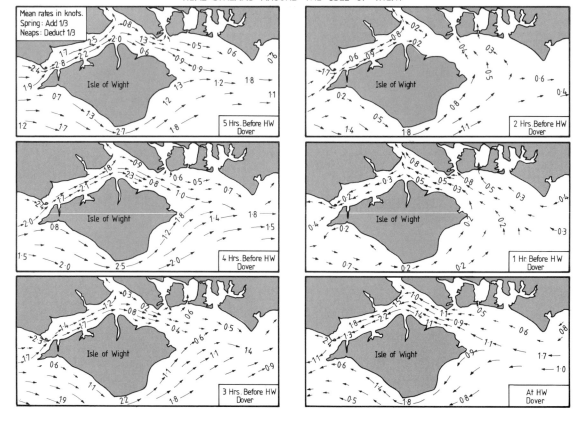

TIDAL STREAMS AROUND THE ISLE OF WIGHT

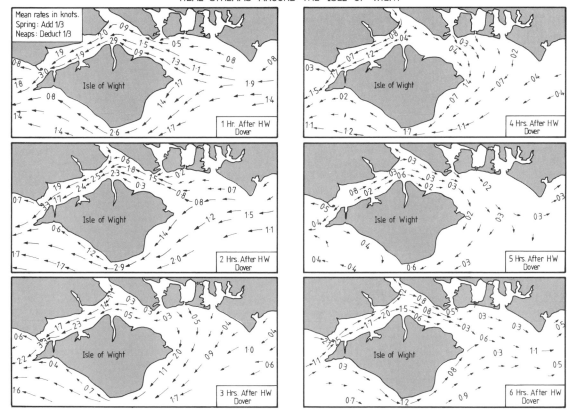

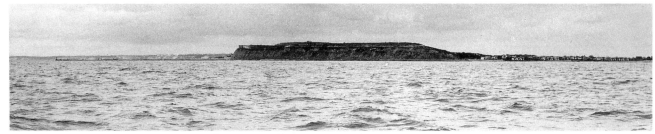

Hengistbury Head *from the south-east. Entrance to Christchurch on right*

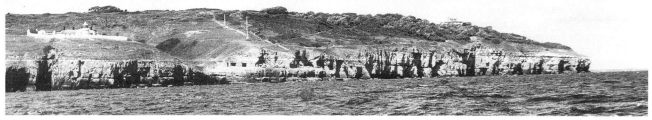

Anvil Point Lighthouse *White tower and squat building 12m high, set 45m above sea-level. Durlston Head to the right*

In the Needles Channel streams in both directions set strongly across the Shingles. Off Hurst Point the north-east stream begins +0505 Dover and the south-west stream at −0055 Dover and attain 4 to 5 knots at springs. Off the Needles the streams tend to be earlier.

In heavy weather the western end of the Isle of Wight should be avoided if possible, especially in south-west winds when it will be worse still if late on the tide after the ebb stream has started. Entry to the Solent under such conditions is safer through the North Channel which lies north of the Shingles, but in gales it is safer still to make for Poole or remain in harbour.

Hengistbury Head   This unlit headland, 5 miles east of Bournemouth pier and 1 mile south-west of the entrance to Christchurch harbour, is of local importance as it is the only headland between the Needles and Handfast Point south of Poole and is conspicuous from seaward. It is composed of dark reddish ironstone, but often appears of a yellowish colour from seaward; the shape is shown in the photograph. There are ledges off the headland and comparatively shoal water as far as Christchurch Ledge $2\frac{1}{2}$ miles south-east of it; the S-cardinal

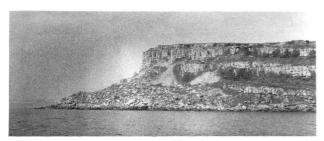

St Alban's Head *from the SSE. No conspicuous buildings*

buoy has been removed. Tidal streams are fairly strong at Springs in the vicinity, and there are overfalls on the ebb tide over the ledges. The streams within Christchurch Bay itself are weak.

Peveril Point to St Alban's Head   There are two recognized tidal races within this area, a small but vicious one off Peveril Point and the larger race off St Alban's Head. There are also local tide rips and under certain conditions patches of rough water may be found practically the whole way from Handfast Point and Old Harry Rocks to St Alban's.

Peveril ledges extend about 3 cables from the low Peveril Point on the south side of Swanage Bay. The depths on the ledges gradually deepen seaward and the end of the reefs is marked by an unlit R can buoy. The tidal streams set straight across the ledges which constitute a danger if a yacht is becalmed. Three cables eastward of Peveril Point the streams are north-north-east +0500 Dover 1½ knots; south-south-west −0215 Dover, 3 knots. In bad weather Peveril Race extends from the Point to seaward of the buoy and especially to the south-east of it during the west-going stream. On a spring ebb tide the rate probably considerably exceeds the rates given.

Durlston Head is a rough headland of a characteristic shape shown on page 28, and is easily identified by the castellated building on its summit. About a mile east-south-east of the headland the north-east-going stream begins +0530 Dover; south-west −0030 Dover; 3 knots Springs.

Inshore Eddy   Between Durlston Head and extending along the Dorset coast westward beyond Lulworth there is an early eddy close inshore contrary to the main English Channel stream farther seaward. The easterly eddy starts about +0400 Dover quickly becoming strong and the westerly about −0200 Dover.

Anvil Point, nearly ½ mile to the south-west of Durlston, is easily located by the conspicuous white lighthouse and white wall round its enclosure which stands above the headland (Fl W 10s. 45m 24M. It also has a VHF lighthouse.

St Alban's Head is the most southerly on this part of the coast and its shape with cliffs at the summit falling into rocks at the base is easily recognized (pic top left). Off St Alban's Head there is a considerable tidal race which lies eastward of the head on the flood tide and westward on the ebb. The race varies considerably in its position and its severity. It extends some 3 miles seaward except during southerly winds when it lies closer inshore. It may be avoided by giving the land a berth of 3 miles. 1½M off the Head the easterly stream begins about +0545 Dover; west −0015 Dover, attaining a rate of between 4 and 5 knots at springs. There is a passage of nearly ½ mile between St Alban's Head and the race but it varies and may be less during onshore winds and is not entirely immune from tidal disturbance. Thus in reasonable weather vessels can avoid the worst of the overfalls by keeping inshore at St Alban's where deep water is found close to the headland. The inshore passage has the advantage of the early fair eddy but a local eddy runs down the west side of St Alban's Head to the south-east nearly continuously.

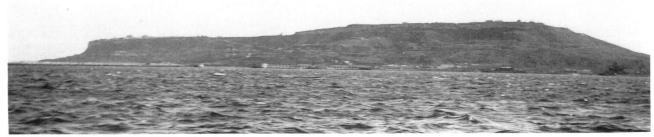

Portland Bill *from the east. Note wedge shape. The Varne at right*

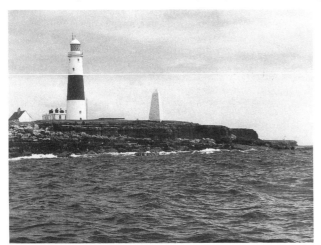

Portland Bill Lighthouse *from the south-west. White tower with red band, 41m high*

Portland Bill and Race   From well seaward Portland has a characteristic shape, appearing like an island, high and broad on its northern end against the low Chesil Beach and sloping down towards the southern end. Here is the round tower with a white and red band lighthouse (Fl (4) W 20s. 43m 29M. Dia 30s.) A 13M FR sector (271°–291°) covers The Shambles shoals for vessels approaching from the E.

Portland Race lies south of Portland Bill, a little to the westward during the ebb and to the eastward during the flood, where in bad weather there is confused and dangerous water so far as and over the whole of the Shambles. The worst part of the Race extends over 2 miles from the Bill and it is well defined by the area of overfalls. At spring tides the Race sometimes attains a rate exceeding 7 knots, but the rate is not uniform and reference is best made to the Admiralty tidal charts around Portland Bill which show hourly details. It may be added that south-west of Portland, during the west-going stream there is a northerly set into West Bay, which at times is strong. When rounding Portland Bill the navigator has two principal options to choose between. The easier one is to pass outside the Race about 3 miles off the Bill in calm or 5 miles in bad weather, especially at spring tides if the wind is against streams.

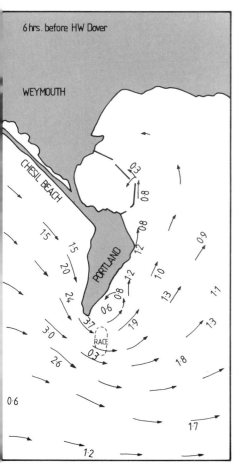
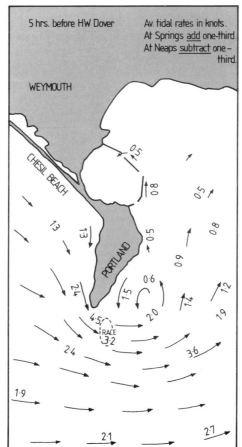
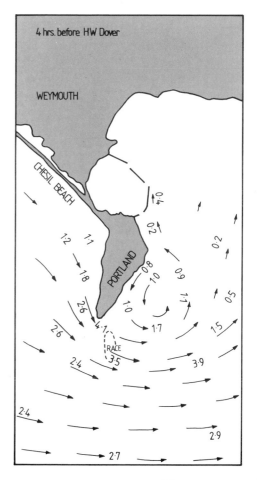

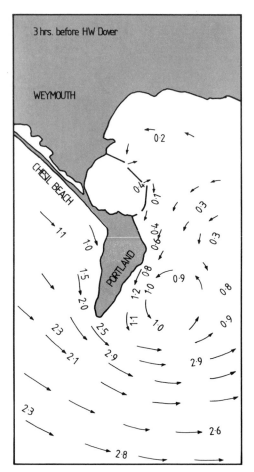

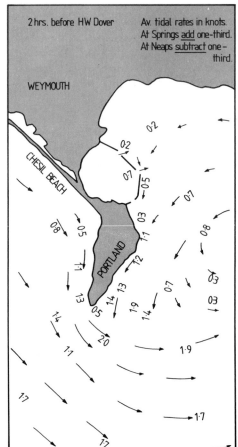

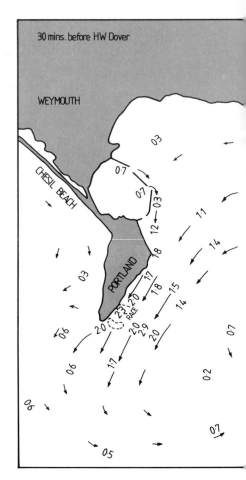

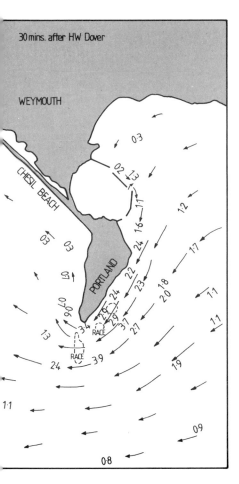

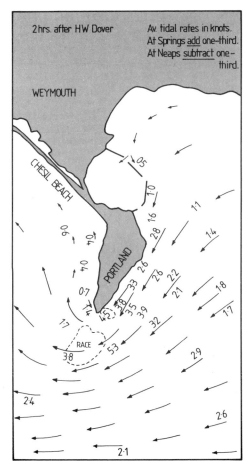

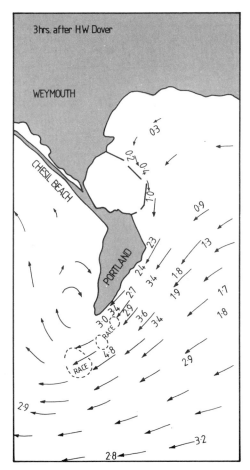

33

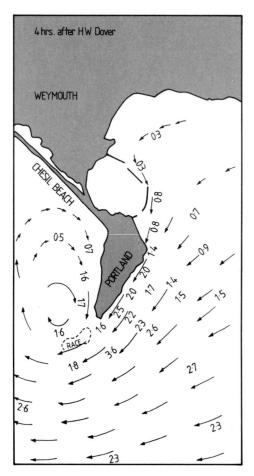

4 hrs. after HW Dover

WEYMOUTH

CHESIL BEACH

PORTLAND

RACE

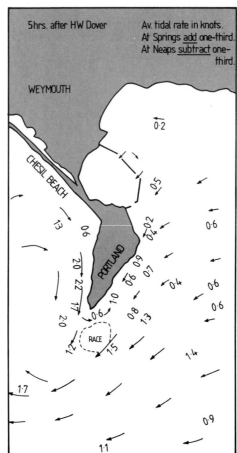

5 hrs. after HW Dover

Av. tidal rate in knots.
At Springs add one-third.
At Neaps subtract one-
third.

WEYMOUTH

CHESIL BEACH

PORTLAND

RACE

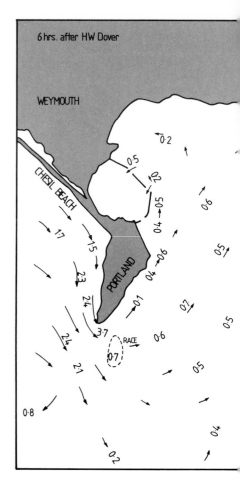

6 hrs. after HW Dover

WEYMOUTH

CHESIL BEACH

PORTLAND

RACE

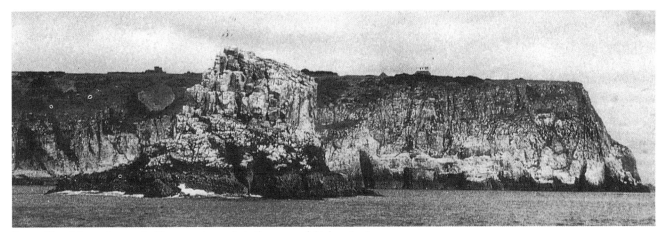

Berry Head *from the south. Note coastguard station near right-hand edge*

The alternative is to use the inner passage which is a channel about ¼ mile wide (varying with direction of wind) which lies between the Bill and the Race. This channel should not be used at night even if ocean-racing navigators do so, and by day only under suitable conditions, for, although the water is comparatively smooth, the streams are strong and the overfalls are not entirely avoided off Grove Point and west of the Bill, according to wind direction. The correct timing of the passage is a matter of the utmost importance.

When bound *westward*, round the Bill between ½ hour before and 2½ hours after HW Dover. When bound *eastward*, round the Bill between 4½ hours after and 5 hours before HW Dover. Whether bound west or east through the inner passage close with Portland at least a mile to the northward of the Bill and

work southward with a fair tide to arrive off the Bill at the correct time.

Golden Cape   A useful landmark 3½ miles east of Lyme Regis and 3 miles west of Bridport. The cape rises to Golden Cap, 186m high, which has pronounced yellow cliffs at its summit which, with sun on them, may be conspicuous from a long distance even in hazy weather. Inshore streams weak.

Beer Head   A conspicuous chalk cliff westward of which lie the red sandstone cliffs of Devon. Inshore streams weak, approximately east +0600 Dover; west at HW Dover.

Berry Head   Bold limestone headland flat topped, with steep end falling at about 45° to the sea. White lighthouse on summit with an elevation of 58m (Fl (2) W 15s). Coastal streams: north +0540 Dover; south −0100 Dover. 1½ knots maximum.

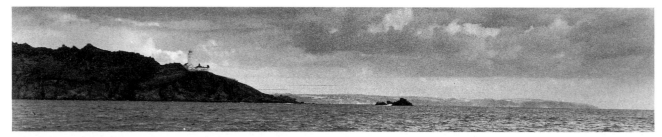

Start Point *from the south-west with unmarked off-lying rocks and Berry Head beyond. White tower 28m high, 62m above sea-level*

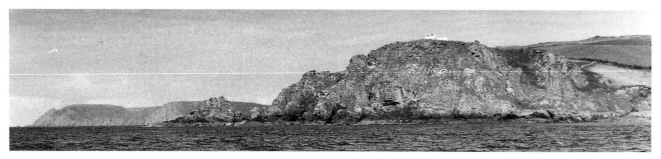

Prawle Point *from the south-east. Prominent old coastguard hut on clifftop 60m above sea-level. Bolt Head beyond (left)*

Charts: BA 442; Im C6; Stan 13

Start Point   A long sharp-ridged headland, with 28m round white lighthouse (Fl (3) W10s. 62m 25M. Horn 60s.) which is unmistakable. A FR 12m Lt. with its arc 210°–255° covers the Skerries bank. There are rocks off the Start which are awash at HW and extend nearly 3 cables south of the Point. The Start race extends nearly a mile seaward of the Point, and its severity depends much on the conditions of wind, tide and swell. The overfalls can be avoided in daylight by passing close to the rocks but there is an outlying one to the south, so care is needed. It is simpler to give the Point a berth of at least a mile. Three miles southward of the Point the streams are: east-north-east +0455 Dover; west-south-west −0120 Dover, about 2 knots Springs. Off Start rocks the streams are about an hour earlier and attain about 4 knots at Springs but are irregular at Neaps.

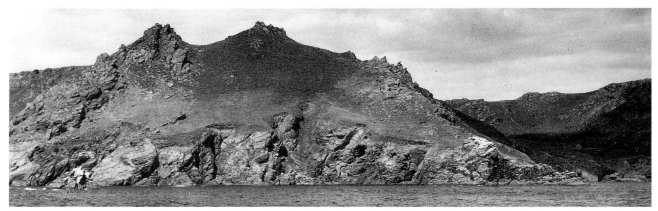

Bolt Head *from the south with Starehole Bay on the right*

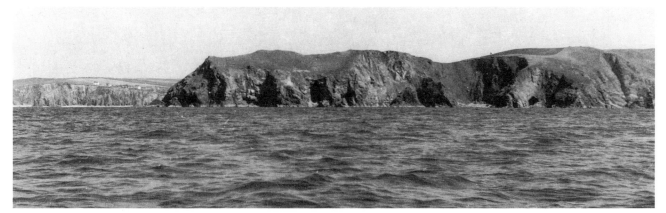

Bolt Tail *from the south-west with Hope Cove on the left*

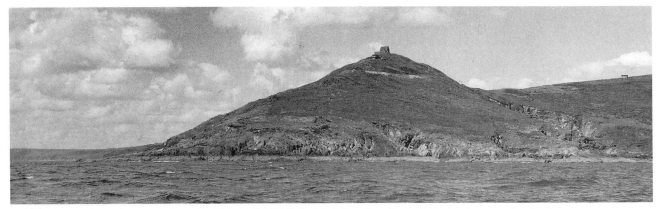

Rame Head *from the south-east, outside Plymouth Sound. Ruined chapel on summit 102m above sea-level*

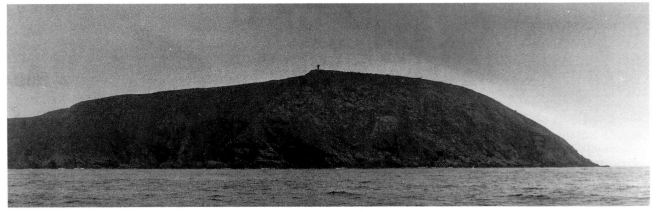

Dodman Point *from the SSW. Stone cross on summit 111m above sea-level. No lighthouse*

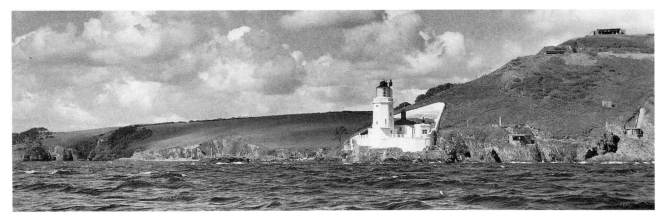

St Anthony's Head *on the eastern side of the entrance to Falmouth. White octagonal tower 19m high*

The next five headlands are all unlit:

Prawle Point This Point lies 3½ miles west of Start Point to the south-east of Salcombe Bar, and has a prominent white Coastguard Station at its summit.

Bolt Head and Bolt Tail Bolt Head stands on the west side of the entrance to Salcombe. The ridge of dark rugged cliffs extending to Bolt Tail is conspicuous.

Rame Head is conspicuous when one is approaching Plymouth Sound. It has a ruined chapel on its summit.

Dodman Point is a most conspicuous headland standing about half-way between Fowey and Falmouth. It is precipitous, 110m high, with a stone cross near south-west extremity. Irregular bottom and tide rips 1½ miles seaward.

St Anthony's Head Lies 9 miles SW of the Dodman, marking the entrance to Falmouth. Its W octagonal tower Lt is OcWR15s. 22m 22M. In fog its horn sounds ev. 30s.

Charts: BA 154; Im C7; Stan 13

Lizard Point The Lizard is a bold headland with conspicuous white buildings and a white wall round their enclosure which stand near its summit. The octagonal tower of the white lighthouse (Fl W 3s. 70m 29M. Siren Mo ('N') 60s.) is situated at the eastern end of the buildings. Six cables to eastward there is a coastguard station and Lloyd's signal station.

The group of rocks known as Stag Rocks, some of which are above water and others dry 4 to 5m, extends over ½ mile south of the Lizard. These can be seen at most states of the tide and avoided, but a mile east of Lizard Point lie the Vrogue Rocks off Bass Point which have less than 2m over them at LW. The Craggan Rocks, with 1m5 over them, lie north-east of Bass Point, but these dangers will be avoided by vessels proceeding east or west to the southward of the Stag Rocks. The Lizard

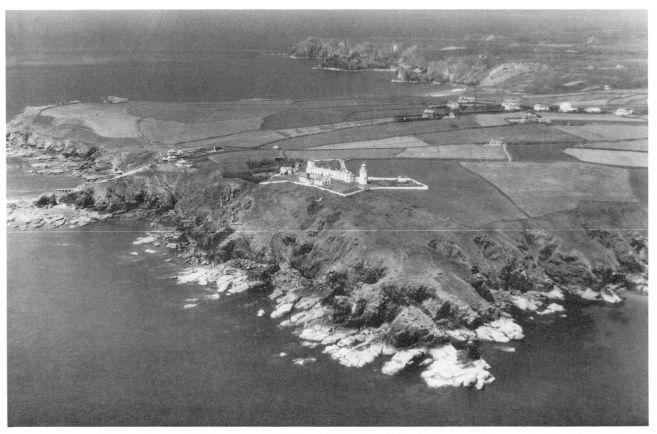

Lizard Point Lighthouse *Octagonal white tower 19m high at right-hand end of buildings, 70m above sea-level, with unmarked off-lying dangers*

Race extends 2 to 3 miles seaward of the Stag Rocks, and at times there is a race south-east of the head. The state of the seas varies considerably according to tide and wind direction, and the seas may be very rough with strong westerly winds against the down-channel stream. Under suitable conditions pass outside the Stag Rocks where the streams start east +0415 Dover; west −0345 Dover. Springs rates are 2 and 3 knots respectively and at times stronger. In rough weather or when a swell is running, especially with wind against a spring tide vessels should keep 3 or more miles off Lizard Point.

Note that the Lizard is the most westerly of the conspicuous headlands on the south coast of England. It is a dividing line in the sense that west of it there is only a limited shelter in Penzance Bay but eastward there are many harbours available in bad weather.

Charts: BA 777; Im C7

Land's End is 20 miles WNW of the Lizard. Although it is higher it is not so conspicuous, due to having no lighthouse on it. The unlit Gwennap Head is its southernmost point, with the dangerous Runnel Stone Rocks running a mile off-shore and marked by a YB south cardinal buoy (Q (6) + LFl 15s.) which has been known to drag off its station in severe weather. In calm weather and with local knowledge it is possible to cut inside, but the distance saved is not worth the ulcers.

The ebb tide sets NW off the point for $9\frac{1}{2}$ hours, starting at HW Dover −0300, and runs up to $2\frac{1}{2}$ knots. The east-going flood turns 6 hours before HW Dover and only runs for three hours.

From the vicinity of the Runnel Stone the Wolf Rock (Fl W 15s. 34m 23M. Dia 30s. Foghorn 30s.) stands out on its own seven miles to the SW, while the Longships Lighthouse 4 miles to the NW (Iso WR 10s. 34m 19M. Horn 15s.) marks the westernmost point of England, excepting the Scilly Isles 20 miles farther west. There are always confused seas around the menacing group of rocks marked by the Longships, and yacht on passage should keep at least a mile to seaward.

Part Two

Harbours and Anchorages

Distances are given in nautical miles, cables and metres.
Bearings and courses are True, to which Variation must be
added and Deviation applied for ship's magnetic compass.

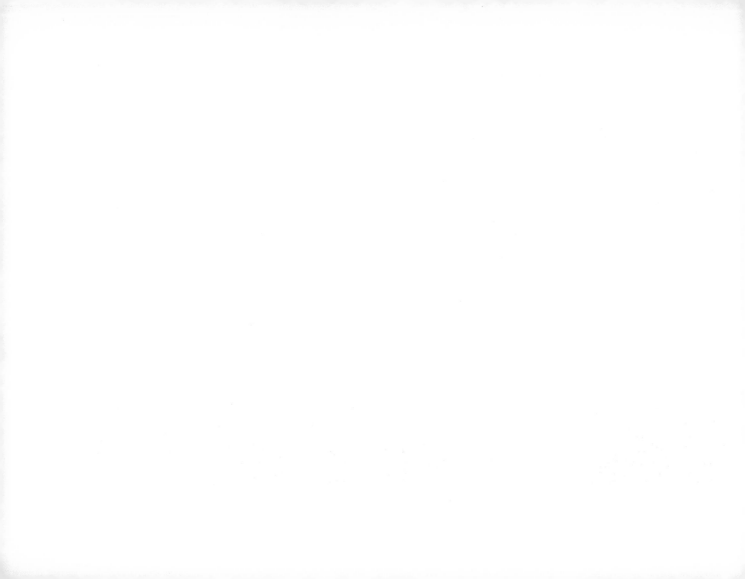

1 Ramsgate

Charts: BA 1827, 1828; Im C8; Stan 9

High Water + *00h. 20m. Dover*
Heights above Datum *MHWS 5m0. MLWS 0m4. MHWN 3m9. MLWN 1m2.*
Depths *Off the entrance the depths are variable outside the new main East-West channel to the RO/RO ferry terminal which passes one cable south of the old breakwater entrance and is dredged to 6m0. The deepest water for entering the Royal Harbour lies close to the West pierhead, where a least depth of 2m3 will be found. On the east side a bar sometimes forms which dries out at LAT. Depths inside the harbour are shown on the plan. The Inner Harbour which forms the marina maintains a constant 3m0 inside the lock-gates, with least depths at its northern end of 2m5.*

RAMSGATE is the only English port in the vicinity of the Straits of Dover offering yachts access and secure alongside berths at all states of the tide. It is a convenient stop-over for yachts making a passage between anywhere in the English Channel and the North Sea.

Its outer harbour is a deepwater port for ferry and container traffic, with a 6m5 approach channel from the east and a dredged 6m5 area inside the new breakwaters which protect the old harbour from all directions. Visiting yachts have the option of lying alongside pontoons inside the W pier or locking into the 600-boat marina.

Approach and Entrance *From the S*, head for the Gull Stream channel, keeping in the W sector of the N Foreland Lt (Fl 5 WR 20s. 57m 21M), a 28m W structure on the cliffs ahead. At the R can S Brake buoy (Fl R (3) 10s.) and the G con W Goodwin buoy (Fl 5s.), keep the bearing of N Foreland Lt Ho W of N(T) and head up the 3.8 miles towards the new E-W ship channel into Ramsgate. The old Ramsgate Channel between

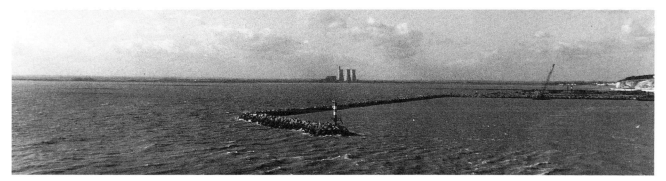

1.1 *West breakwater head with Richborough cooling towers beyond*

45

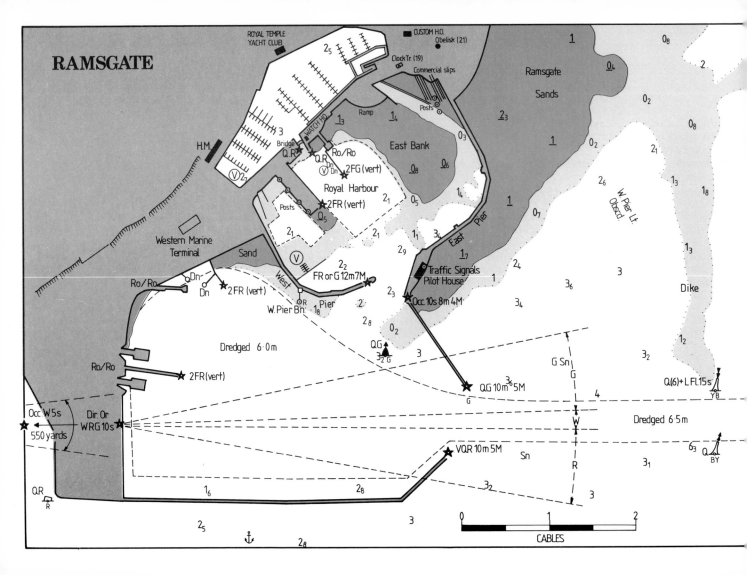

RAMSGATE

ROYAL TEMPLE
YACHT CLUB

CUSTOM H.O.
Obelisk (21)

Clock Tr. (19)

Commercial slips

Ramsgate
Sands

2_5

WATCH H.O.

1_3

1_4

Ramp

Posts

3

H.M.

Bridge

Q.R.

Ro/Ro

East Bank

2_3

0_3

1

0_8

$(V) 2_1$

Q.R.
Dn
(V) Dn

2FG (vert)

Royal Harbour

0_8

0_6

0_2

0_8

2_1

Western Marine
Terminal

Posts

2FR (vert)

Q_5

2_1

0_5

1_4

2_1

1

0_7

2_6

2_1

1_3

1_8

W. Pier Lt.
Obscd.

1_3

Sand

(V)

2_1

2_1

1_1

3_4

East Pier

1

2_9

1_7

2_4

3

Dike

Ro/Ro

Dn

Dn

2FR (vert)

West

FR or G 12m 7M

2_2

2_3

Traffic Signals
Pilot House

Occ 10s 8m 4M

3_6

3_4

1_2

W. Pier Bn

R

Pier

1_8

2

2_8

0_2

3

3_2

Dredged 6·0 m

QG
$3_2 G$

3

3_4

3

G Sn

QG 10m 5M

3_6

G

4

Q(6)+L Fl.15s

YB

Ro/Ro

2FR(vert)

W

Dredged 6·5m

Occ W 5s

Dir. Or
WRG 10s

VQR 10m 5M

Sn

R

3_1

6_3 Q

BY

550 yards

3_2

3

Q.R.

R

1_6

2_8

3

3_2

2_5

⚓

2_8

0   1   2

CABLES

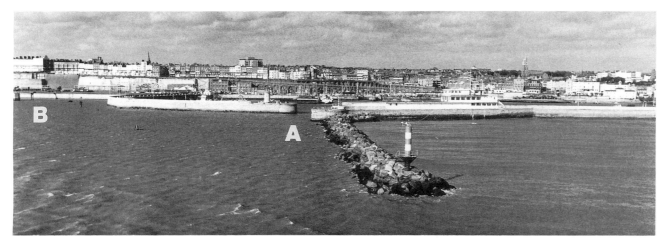

1.2 *(A) East breakwater head with entrance to Royal Harbour (B) Ferry harbour*

Sandwich Flats to the W and the Brake sand on the E is now only useful as an approach to the Pegwell Bay channel into Sandwich.

The E-cardinal BYB E Brake buoy (Q (3) 10s.) lies 1.8 miles due E of the new harbour entrance. It is perfectly in order to leave it on either side, so long as you observe the unlit BY N-cardinal Quern buoy by leaving it to port. By night a transit of 294½° on the E pierhead (Oc 10s. 8m 9M) and the W pierhead (FR or G 12m 7M) will bring you in on a safe course. Leaving the Quern buoy head WNW to pass through the new breakwater entrance (see plan). Once inside swing slowly to starboard, keeping at least 100 yards SW of the new North Breakwater, leaving to port the G con Harbour buoy (QG).

Approaching from the N or E, pass close to seaward of the Broadstairs Knoll R can buoy (Fl R 2.5s.) 1½ miles due E of the cliffs on a WSW course until picking up the fairway as described above.

Tidal Currents and Signals   Off the breakwater entrance the tidal stream sets to the NNE at over 2 knots at Springs from HW Dover for five hours; it runs to the SSW from HW Dover +6h. until 1 h. before the next HW. A tidal light at the end of W Pier shows the depths of water at the entrance to Royal Harbour: FR indicates more than 3mo depth; FG when less than 3mo.

Traffic Signals   IALA Port Traffic Signals are displayed near W pierhead.

Lights   The new W ferry terminal RO/RO berths have a Dir Oc WRG 10s. light with a 2° W centred on the leading course along the fairway from seaward of 270°. The breakwater

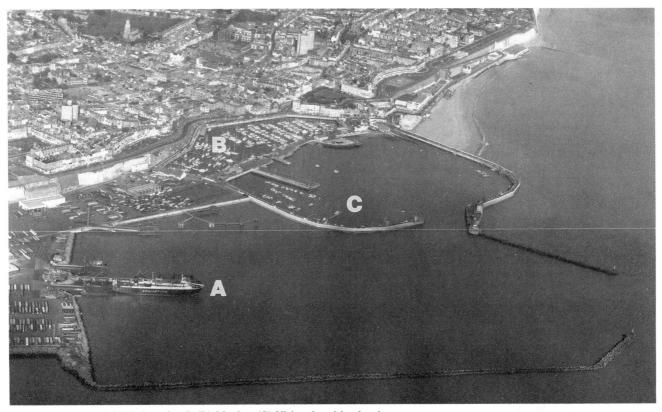

1.3 *Ramsgate. (A) RO/RO ferry berth (B) Marina (C) Visitors' waiting berths*

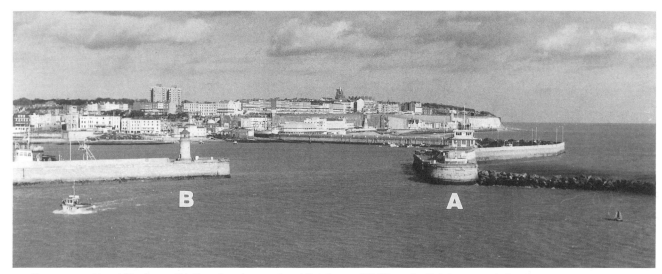

1.4 *Entrance to Royal Harbour. (A) East breakwater head lighthouse (B) West pier lighthouse and signals*

entrance has Bns marking either side: G with VQ G to starboard, opposite R with VQ R to port. The old W pierhead has an 11m round granite tower (see pic 1.4) with a F R or G 12m 7M. The colour of the light indicates depth in the entrance to Royal Harbour: FR says there is over 3m; FG means less. The E pierhead opposite has a 4m R and W metal column with Oc W 10s. 10m 5M Lt on it. Other Lts in the harbour as on plan, with entrance to the marina governed by its own IALA light signals. A single R light beside the gate means that it is not due to open.

Anchorage and Berthing   No anchoring is allowed inside the harbour, but in favourable conditions yachts can anchor in Pegwell Bay close S of the new outer breakwater. For berths inside the Royal Harbour contact the HM on Ch 16 or 14 or by communicating with the Dockmaster from his office on the E side of the lock-gates. Yachts may be hailed by the watch-house on E pierhead and told to lie by the W pier in 1m7 or alongside the E pier in 2m0. The HM can also be contacted by phone on Thanet (0843) 592277–9. Customs are on (0843) 593501.

Facilities   Water at all piers. Fuel, chandlery, repairs and shore power in the marina. Slipway in Royal Harbour. All the amenities of a major holiday port. Royal Temple YC overlooks marina.

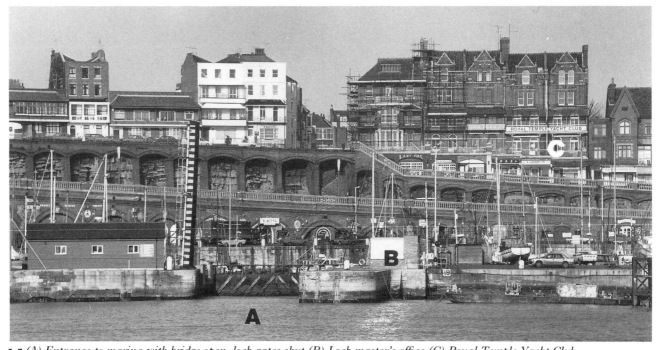

1.5 *(A) Entrance to marina with bridge open, lock-gates shut (B) Lock-master's office (C) Royal Temple Yacht Club*

Weather   BBC shipping forecast area: Dover/Thames.
Marine call tel: 0898–500456.
London Weather Centre tel: 071–836 4311.
BBC Radio London: 1458 kHz 94.9 MHz at 0714,
0814, 1300, 1714; Sat–Sun 0800.

Radio Kent on 1035 or 774 kHz or 96.7 MHz at intervals between 0603 and 1806 (1305 at weekends).
North Foreland Shipping Weather on Ch 26 0803 and 2003.

*2 Sandwich

Charts: BA 1827; Im C8; Stan 9

High Water *at bar +ooh. 15m. Dover.*
Heights above Datum *Richborough: MHWS 3m7. MHWN 2m6. Bar dries at LW.*
Tides *The ebb runs for 7 hours and the flood for 5 hours at Sandwich Town.*

Depths *On the bar dries om3 to om9 at CD. Entrance channel and river shallow. At HW Springs navigable with a maximum draught of about 4m5 or about 3m0 at Neaps as far as Sandwich.*

SANDWICH lies 4½ miles from the mouth of the meandering River Stour, once the channel for great fleets heading out to sea from one of the original Cinque Ports charged with the defence of the realm against invaders since Norman times. In the 18th century the local earl launched the fast-food business with

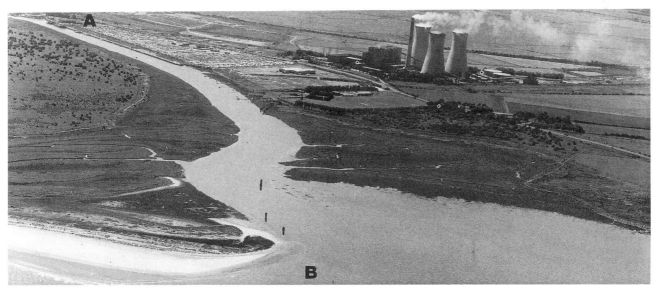

2.1 *Mouth of River Stour. (A) Commercial berths (B) Channel beacons with topmarks*

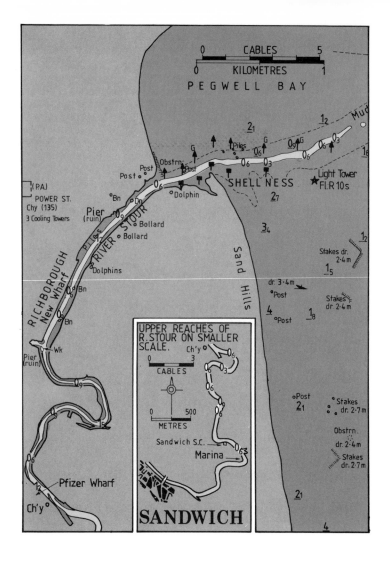

sandwiches devoured during non-stop sessions at the gaming tables. In our times its golf links gave Ian Fleming the inspiration for some of James Bond's rougher matches. Nowadays yachts lie alongside the Town Quay.

Approach The Stour runs into the SW corner of Pegwell Bay, about 2 miles SW of Ramsgate. The three cooling towers alongside the 135m chimney of the power station are conspicuous from miles away. The bay dries out except for a narrow, shifting channel carrying the river water. At its seaward end the channel is marked by R and G buoys. Halfway along a red framework tower (Fl R 10s. 3m 4M) which has to be left close to port marks the start of the inshore end of the channel. This is marked by R and G posts with topmarks. Approach only in good weather by day, preferably 2½ h. before HW. From Ramsgate steer SW to the buoyed channel and then stay in the middle, especially once inside the river itself.

The town bridge can be opened at 24-hours' notice; thereafter there are 12 miles of navigable water for boats of up to 1m2 draught. The entrance channel and lower reaches are navigable about 2½ h. either side of HW for draught of 1m2. Just inside the river entrance is a dolphin on the port hand, with a pole and diamond topmark.

Berthing It is not practicable to anchor anywhere in the river. One mile downstream from Sandwich there is a marina with 60 pontoon berths, most of which dry out. Here at HW Springs there is 2m4, down to 1m8 at MLWN. The river becomes narrower and very congested in this reach owing to numerous moorings. Farther downstream Richborough Wharf is private, used by the tankers feeding the power station. There is another small commercial wharf a short distance upstream. At Sandwich the bottom is hard chalk covered by a very thin layer of mud. For deep-draught yachts it is wise to make preparations for drying out by the wall.

Facilities Sandwich Sailing and Motor Boat Club, Bayside

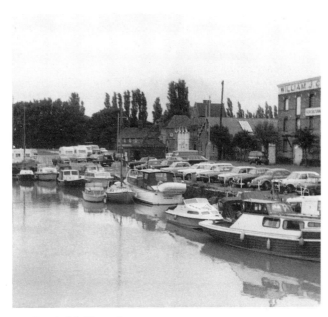

2.2 *Sandwich Town Quay*

Marine yard and most facilities at marina; tel. 0304–613335.
Water at Sandwich Town Quay on application to the Quay-
master (tel. 613283). Petrol at garage near quay. Shops. EC
Wed. Hotels. Yacht yard above bridge. Sandwich MBC near
marina has a slip.
   Weather   See Ramsgate p. 50.

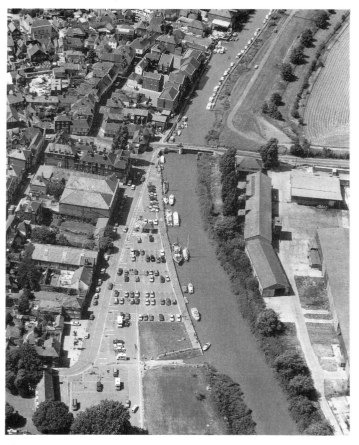

2.3 *Town bridge and upper reaches of River Stour*

3 Dover

Charts: BA 1698; Im C8; Stan 9

Heights above Datum *MHWS 6m9. MLWS 0m8. MHWN 5m3. MLWN 2m0; but irregular, depending on wind conditions.*
Depths *Dover is a large artificial harbour divided into two parts. The big expanse of the outer harbour is a deep-water port. The inner western part between the Admiralty pier and the Prince of Wales pier has about 5m in the entrance, but the depths gradually reduce towards the inner tidal harbour, which dries out at MLWS at its northern arm. Beyond this are the inner basins: Wellington Dock, which is used by yachts, has 4m5 at Springs, 3m3 Neaps. Granville Dock is deep.*

DOVER is the busiest port in England. Owing to its heavy commercial traffic yachtsmen are not encouraged to use the harbour unless they obey the traffic control signals implicitly. They are only welcome to stay for a maximum of two weeks in the Wellington Dock during April–September. These are the only alongside berths in the harbour available to yachts. Boats which anchor off may not be left untended.

Approach and Entrance Dover harbour is some 2 miles SW of the S Foreland. By day the long breakwaters overlooked by the famous Castle make the harbour easy to identify. At night the breakwater lights are: The W Entrance has Oc R 30s. 21m 18M on S breakwater and Fl 7.5s. 21m 20M at the seaward end of Admiralty Pier. It has a diaphone fog signal 10s. and displays the Port movement Lts. Towards the E Entrance the Knuckle Lt is Oc WR 10s. 15m 15M with an F Y 17m 4M at the entrance. The E Arm has Port Control and a fog signal Dia (2) 30s. Lts inside as shown on plan.

Yachts are required to use the western entrance, owing to the much heavier commercial traffic using the eastern one. *A careful look-out should be kept for the entry signals.* Permission to enter may also be requested by Aldis lamp or International Code signals (SV: I wish to enter; SW: I wish to leave); yachts with VHF call Dover Port Control on Ch 74 or on Ch 16 to establish a working frequency (usually Ch 12). A series of short flashes from Port Control on Admiralty Pier indicates: 'STOP–WAIT'.

All yachts should keep well clear of the actual entrances until the moment they receive their entry or exit signals, in order to leave room for bigger ships to manoeuvre or swing round just inside the entrances. Local tidal streams vary considerably and attain their maximum Spring rate of 3 knots. Flood sets NE at HW − 1 to +3 h. Always enter under power if possible.

Traffic Signals covering both entrances are exhibited at the ends of the Eastern Arm and Admiralty Pier. All traffic is regulated by day or night by IALA port signals using directional high-intensity lights beamed to seaward or inshore, depending on whom they apply. Signals are vertically displayed, as follows (see inside back cover):

RRR Flashing	Emergency. Entrance closed.	
RRR Fixed	Entry or exit prohibited from the direction indicated.	
GWG	Ships may proceed to or from direction indicated.	

Navigation in Outer Harbour The Harbour Patrol launch will be found in the outer harbour. When it shows a Fl Bu light by night it will act as a radio relay. Any instructions given from it must be observed. Yachts should beware of hovercraft and jetfoils who may use either entrance at 40 knots. They must keep well clear of Channel ferries and cargo ships manoeuvring in the fairway.

Inner Harbour Anchorage is not permitted between Admiralty and Prince of Wales Piers. The Granville Dock is not available to yachts. Permission should be asked of Dockmaster

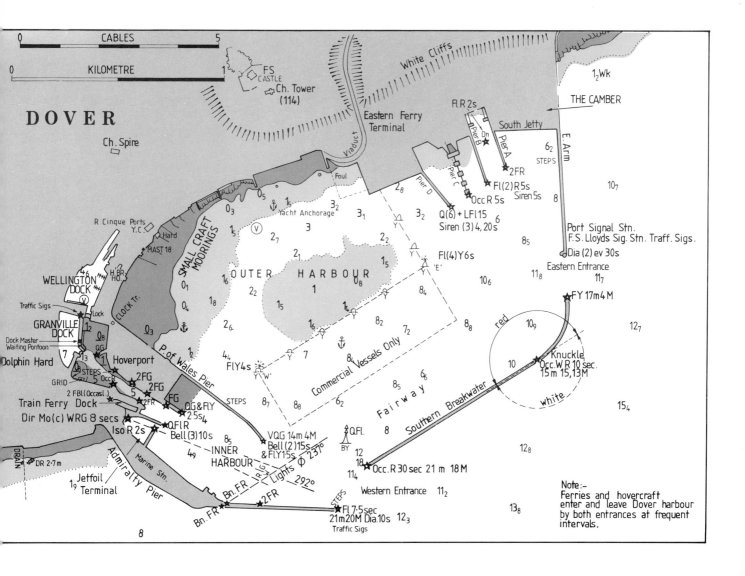

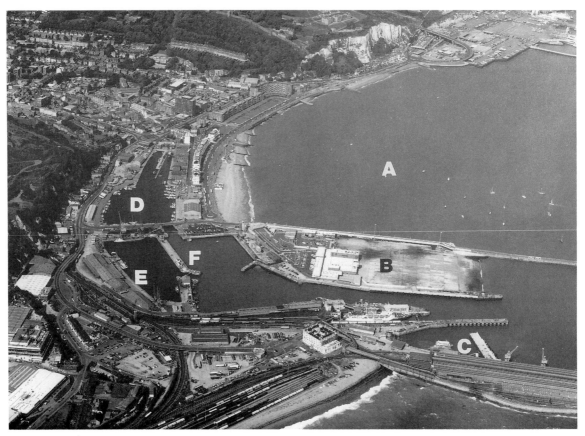

3.1 *Western end of Dover Harbour. (A) Yacht moorings (B) Hoverport (C) Jetfoil terminal (D) Yacht harbour in Wellington Docks (E) Granville Docks (commercial) (F) Dockmaster's office*

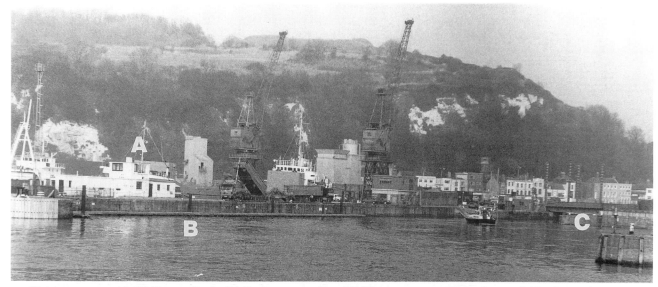

3.2 *Waiting area outside Wellington Dock. (A) Dockmaster's office (B) Waiting pontoon (C) Lock open, bridge lowered*

or the Harbour launch to lie alongside the waiting pontoon next to his office until lock-gates open to enter Wellington Dock, usually between 1½ h. before HW to 1 h. after. Dockmaster's office manned – 2½ h. HW to +1 h. Tel: 0304–206560, ex 4531.

Wellington Dock Signals exhibited from top of 9mo tower on west side of dock entrance. *By Day and Night* – IALA Port Movement Lts as described above.

A Fl amber light is shown 5 minutes before the bridge is swung.

Craft intending to leave Wellington Dock must inform the Dockmaster's office beforehand by visiting him at the entrance of the tidal Harbour next to waiting pontoon. Clearance to sail is given after settling harbour dues.

Jetfoil Terminal is inshore of the new breakwater running NNE of the BR Marine Station. Its entrance is on a directional light 292° Mo (C) WRG 8s.

Anchorage E of Prince of Wales Pier, as near to the shore as soundings permit. The Royal Cinque Ports YC has one visitors' mooring which may be used by yachts. Private moorings off the club may not be picked up without prior permission from the club (tel. 0304–206262). Yachts are not permitted to use the Camber or Eastern Docks. Inside Wellington Dock on the pontoon immediately to port of the lock-gate (NOT on the pontoons at the E wall), or as directed.

Facilities Harbour Office (tel. 0304–240400). Customs (0304–202441). Water showers and WCs at Wellington Dock or by courtesy at yacht club, which offers temporary membership to visiting yachts. Chandlery, fuel and stores available. EC Wed. Scrubbing and minor repairs at Dolphin Hard by arrangement at Dockmaster's office. Yacht club: R. Cinque Ports YC. Launching site: from beach below centre promenade, boats up to 4m8 long. Car park. Two stations, fast trains to London. Buses to all parts.

Weather See Ramsgate p. 50.
Navigation warnings by CG on Ch 16, 69, 11 or 80 for information. Ch 11 at 40 and 55 m. past the hour in poor visibility.

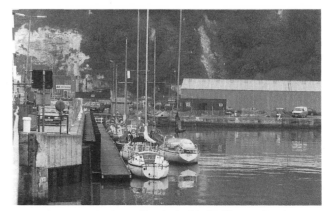

3.3 *Pontoon berths immediately inside Wellington Dock, generally assigned to visitors*

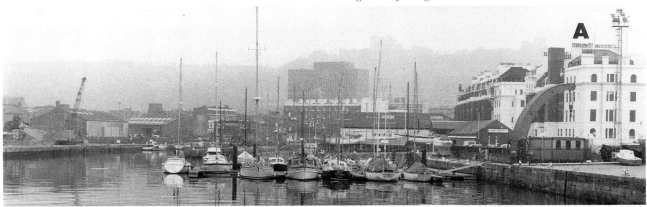

3.4 *Wellington Dock, mostly for long-term berth-holders. (A) Dover Harbour Board offices*

*4 Folkestone

Charts: BA 1991; Im C8; Stan 9

High Water *ooh. 12m. Dover.*
Heights above Datum *MHWS 7m1. MLWS om7. MHWN 5m7. MLWN 2mo.*
Depths *The outer harbour is dredged to a least depth of 4m5 and is formed by the breakwater which extends into deep water. In the entrance to the inner harbour there is 5m5 at MHWS and from 3m3 to 4m2 MHWS within the harbour, and at Neaps 1mo less. At LW it dries out everywhere.*

FOLKESTONE is mainly a commercial port with its RO/RO ferry terminal. The inner harbour is only suitable for yachts with legs or those prepared to dry out by the rough wall at the E pier. It is not a good refuge in bad weather and yachts are only welcome for occasional overnight moorings, as the whole inner harbour is full up. The inner harbour faces E but the entrance itself receives extra protection from the west by a long breakwater built for British Rail ferries and which forms the outer harbour. The inner harbour is mostly used by fishing boats equipped with legs. The town itself has all the facilities of a summer holiday resort.

Approach and Entrance Folkestone is about 5½ miles westward of Dover and is the largest town on the coast between Dungeness and the Foreland. The town is thus easy to recognize and the harbour lies nearer its eastern end, behind a conspicuous outer breakwater. There are rocky ledges to the west of the breakwater and east of the inner harbour entrance. Of these the Mole Head Rocks, less than 2 cables east of the inner end of the

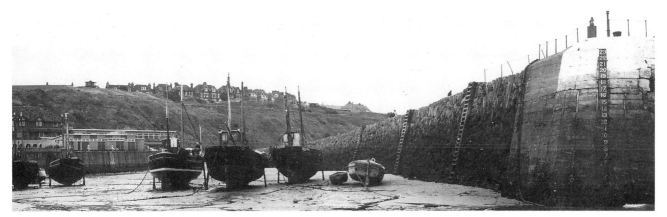

4.1 *Inner harbour at low water*

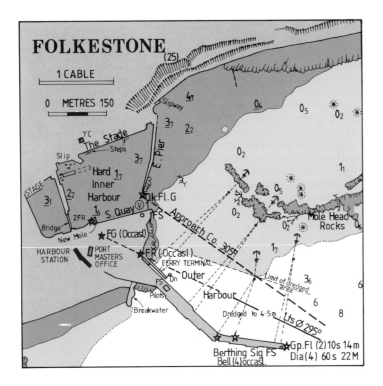

to recognize and the harbour lies nearer its eastern end, behind
a conspicuous outer breakwater. There are rocky ledges to the
west of the breakwater and east of the inner harbour entrance.
Of these the Mole Head Rocks, less than 2 cables east of the
inner end of the outer breakwater, and the ledges off Copt

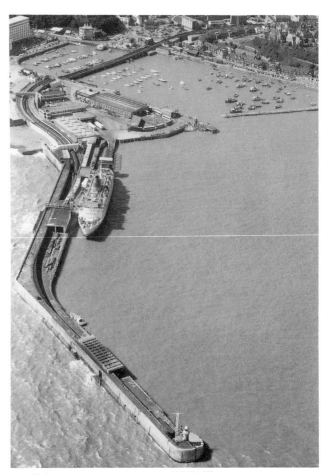

4.2 *Folkestone at high water*

outer breakwater, and the ledges off Copt Point are the more dangerous. To clear these when approaching from the east keep the S Foreland well open of the Dover cliffs. Eddy on east stream. Then when the south end of the east pier (Q G) of the inner harbour bears 305° alter course leaving the outer breakwater close to port. Watch for tidal streams running up to 2 knots off pierhead: ENE from HW Dover −2 h.; setting WSW from Dover +3½ h. Make allowance for the fact that it shoals about 2 cables off the inner harbour and shelves gradually to −1mo at the entrance. For depths within the harbour see *Anchorage and Harbour*.

Signals at the outer end of the new ferry pier are shown for car ferries by means of a black flag or 1, 2 or 3 spherical shapes.

Lights, etc. Outer breakwater Gp Fl W (2) 10 s. 14m 22M. Fog dia (4) 60s. E pierhead Q G Occas. Two F R on mole at south quay when commercial vessel about to enter.

Anchorage and Harbour

(1) Anchorage outside the inner harbour is inadvisable owing to the ferry traffic and risk of fouling the ground moorings and long chains used for winching off the ferries. It is also exposed and has indifferent holding ground. No yacht may *ever* moor alongside the ferry pier except in dire emergency. (2) Yachts may lie in the inner harbour if there is room inside the E pier on legs or alongside the pier. At LAT the harbour dries 1mo at the entrance, about 2m2 in the centre and up to 3m7 at the northern end of the E pier. Yachtsmen must calculate the tide level by reference to the heights above datum at the head of the chapter, but boats up to 1m5 draught can enter 3 hours either side of HW. The swing bridge at western end of inner harbour is permanently fixed and the shallow inner basin (controlled by Folkestone Corporation) can be entered only by boats able to pass below it.

Facilities Water at quay. Good shopping centre. EC Wed. Station. Buses to all parts. Yacht club: Folkestone SC near slipway in inner harbour. HM tel. 0303–54947. VHF Ch 11 or 16; Customs 0303–54604.

Weather See Ramsgate p. 50.
Shipping forecast area: Dover.
Navigation Warnings: see Dover p. 58.

*5 Rye

Charts: BA 1991; Im C8; Stan 9

High Water *at entrance – ooh. o5m. Dover.*
Heights above Datum *near approach: MHWS 7m7.
MHWN 6mo. Dries LW. Harbour MHWS 5m3. MHWN 3m6.*
Depths *In the channel there is only a fresh-water trickle at
MLWS. At MHWS there is about 3m4 to 4m5 in the harbour
alongside the catwalk staging and 1m6 to 2m8 at MHWN.*

RYE HARBOUR is ¾ mile from the entrance of the River Rother,
and is a small village. The town itself is another 2 miles up the
river which is navigable at HW and is increasingly used by cargo
vessels; it is one of the Cinque Ports and so charming that it
attracts many visitors. There are good hotels and restaurants.
Rye Harbour has a bad reputation due to its shifting entrance
and the loss of the lifeboat crew W of the entrance in 1928.
However, the entrance is clearly marked. Given an offshore
wind and fair weather and the right state of tide, strangers
should not find the entrance unduly difficult. A SW wind Force
5 is definitely uncomfortable and probably too much for a first
attempt. Power is desirable as the tide runs very hard in the
narrow channel – the flood is stronger than the ebb, which is
unusual in rivers.

Approach and Entrance The entrance lies at the apex of
Rye Bay. From the eastward follow the low coast from Dungeness for some 7 miles keeping about a mile offshore until
reaching the RW Rye Fairway safe-water buoy (Fl 10s.) 1.8
miles SE of the conspicuous west pier and the tripod beacon.
Westward of the entrance the shore is also low (but hills behind)
for a distance of 5 miles to Fairlight, which is high and can be

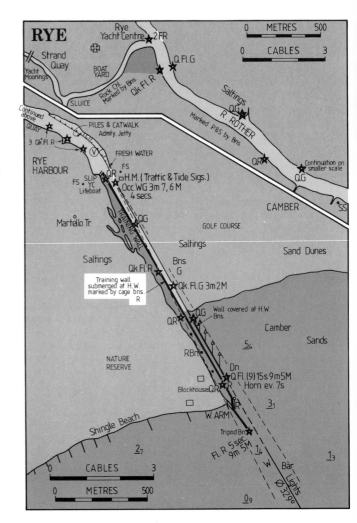

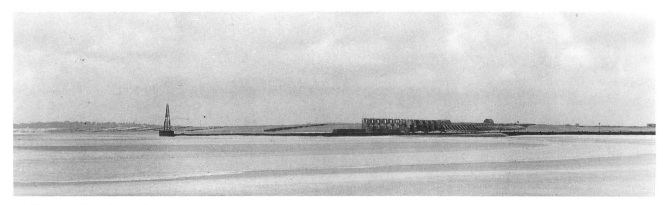

5.1 *Entrance from the south-east at low water*

recognized by the square tower of the church, and its coastguard station.

The entrance and channel to Rye Harbour, from 30 to 45m wide, lie between the E and W piers. On the W side a long training wall has a groyne which extends to seaward of the entrance. This training wall is covered between half tide and HW (depths above 2m4), and it is marked by a series of pole bns with cage topmarks some on top of dolphins; three Q R Lts at night placed at irregular intervals along the walls as far as Rye Harbour and three Fl R Lts at the bend beyond it. At its seaward extremity there stands a tripod Lt dolphin Fl R 5 s. 7m 6M. The east pier is also long, though it does not extend as far seaward; at its end there is a Lt post Q (9) 15 s. 7m 5M with a Q G three cables NW where the E bank begins. At MHWS the tops of this E pier are just showing, but it is marked by two posts with con topmarks.

Vessels making for Rye should head up towards the Rye Fairway buoy, then alter course to 335° so as to leave the wood tripod of the W pier open on the port bow. There is always an easterly set across the harbour entrance, especially on the flood tide. Within the entrance a course mid-channel is possibly the best to take, although the deeper water is on the W side. However, care must be taken on the flood when side currents flowing across the training wall may affect steering. The cage beacons are fixed to the *inside* edge of the training wall except for one off the HM's office – a prominent solitary house on the east bank of the Rother opposite the lifeboat slip.

The entrance should not be approached by vessels with a draught of 2m earlier than 3 h. before HW; the best time to enter is from 1 h. before HW; the best time to leave is not later than 1 h. after HW (but for yachts of moderate draught 2½ h. either side is possible with care at Springs). A tide gauge is fitted to the seaward end of the eastern training wall.

Tidal Signals are shown by day from a mast just behind the

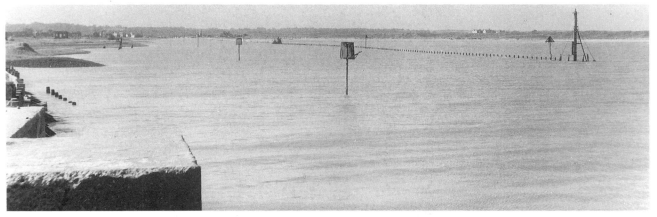

5.2 *Porthand red cages mark submerged training wall off the west bank*

Harbour Office, about ¾ mile within the entrance on the E side, and by night from the roof of the Office when any merchant ship (irrespective of size) is expected, but the signals are hard to see in poor visibility. Depths over bar: 2m4 to 3m0, a G light; over 3m0, a R light.

Traffic Signals   When a cargo vessel is moving in the harbour a B ball is hoisted by day or an amber Q Lt is exhibited on HO at night; all vessels must give way.

Lights, etc.   From Bn on western arm extension Fl R 5s. 7m 6M; on eastern pier end Q (9) ev 15s. 7m 5M. Lts on east side of channel leading up the channel at 329°: front, Q G; rear, Oc W G with W sector 326.5°–331.5° Q R on Bns or dolphins on W side of channel as previously referred to. Fog dia on western arm extension.

From the Harbour up-river the banks are marked by beacons with Q G and Q R lights leading to 2F R (vert) where the Rother joins the Brede in the heart of the old town.

Anchorage and Berths   In fair weather yachts awaiting the tide for Rye should anchor close to Rye Fairway buoy (where there is a least depth of 5m9). In W or SW winds yachts should anchor behind Dungeness, close to the Coastguard's House. With sufficient rise of tide all visiting yachts should moor at special berths provided alongside the piles at Rye Harbour village, about a mile from the entrance on the E side of the river, just beyond the HM's Office. This is about 2 miles from Rye town. The berths are lighted at night. Double mooring is not allowed. Care should be taken when turning at Rye Harbour village at Springs.

The large range of tide calls for careful mooring, as winds blowing on to the staging have been the cause of many broken

64

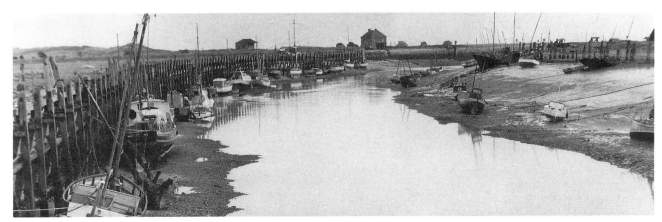

5.3 *Looking downstream at low water. Harbour Office at end of staging*

masts or damaged spreaders. Yachts will lie afloat for about 4 hours, then take the bottom, which is hard muddy shingle. A vacant berth may indicate wreckage below water – always consult the HM, who can be contacted on VHF Ch 16.

The river is navigable for craft drawing up to 2m7 at MHWS as far as Strand Quay in the heart of the historic old town of Rye, where drying-alongside berths or moorings may be found by prior arrangement. Consult the HM before heading upstream.

Facilities Water is available from a hose-pipe at the S end of catwalk staging – apply to HM (tel. 0797–225225) at Strand Quay or on Ch 16 or 14. Hose-pipe at corner of catwalk above visitor's berth. Stores at Rye town 2 miles away (3.2 km) or (limited) in Rye Harbour where there is a chandlery or at a caravan site south of village by the Martello tower. EC Tues. PO

at harbour and town. Small boat-builders. Launching site: slip with road access at Rye Harbour village, but is only usable for a few hours either side of HW (a power cable marked by beacons runs across near here to the lighthouse). Yacht club: Rye Harbour SC on the opposite bank to the HO. Good bus service from the harbour village to the town where there are rail and bus connections to all parts. Excellent shopping. Customs are in the town (tel. 0797-223110).

Weather See Ramsgate p. 50.

BBC shipping forecast area Dover/Wight

Radio Sussex 1485 kHz at 0600, 0630, 0700, 0730, 0800, 0830, thence on the hour. (Weekends on the hour.)

6 Newhaven

Charts: BA 2154; Im C9; Stan 9

High Water   *ooh. 13m. Dover.*
Heights above Datum   *MHWS 6m6. MLWS om6. MHWN 5m2. MLWN 1m9.*
Depths   *Dredged to 5m5 in the entrance, along East Wharf to Sleeper's Hole, 3m5 up to west side Ballast Wharf and not less than 1m2 to bridge leading to R. Ouse. Silting and dredging continually occurring.*

NEWHAVEN is primarily a commercial port but it also offers good facilities for yachts in the marina dredged out of the W bank. The town itself is not interesting, but the distance by bus to Seaford or Eastbourne is short, and there are pleasant walks if weather-bound. There is a regular ferry service to Dieppe.

Approach and Entrance   Newhaven harbour lies at the mouth of the R. Ouse just over 7 miles W of Beachy Head, and 3 miles W of Seaford Head. The town of Seaford is 5 miles westward of Beachy Head and for some 2 miles W of Seaford the shore is low and shingly. At the western end of Seaford Bay is Burrow Head, and just eastward at the foot of this is Newhaven. The big breakwater at the entrance is conspicuous and makes an easily recognizable landmark.

From the eastward stand well away from Seaford Head and steer for position off Burrow Head. Alter course when the entrance bears N, and leave to the westward the outer breakwater, steering in towards the E pier, which is some 3 cables away. In bad weather, with an onshore wind, there is an awkward sea off the entrance S of the breakwater. Steer up mid-channel observing signals shown at southern end of N pier. Within ½ mile of shore, weak W-going stream starts about 1½ to 2

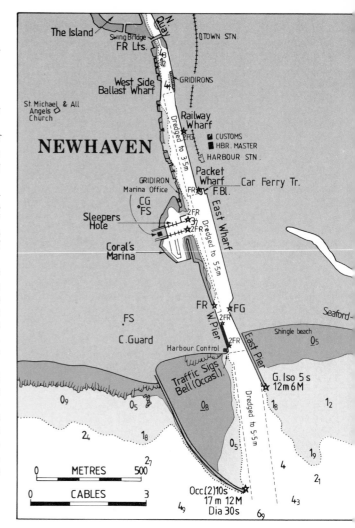

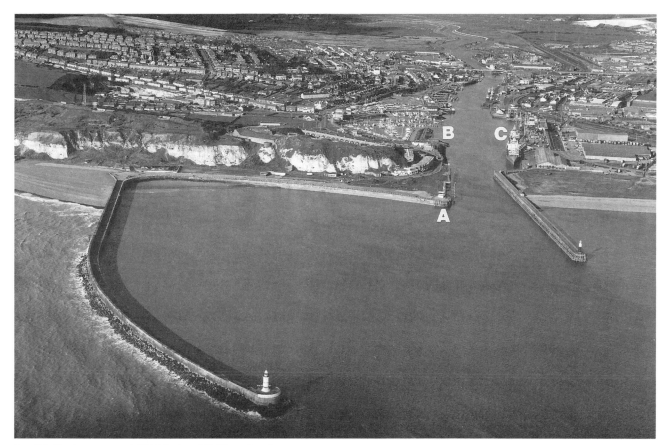

6.1 *(A) Harbour control (B) Marina (C) Ferry berths*

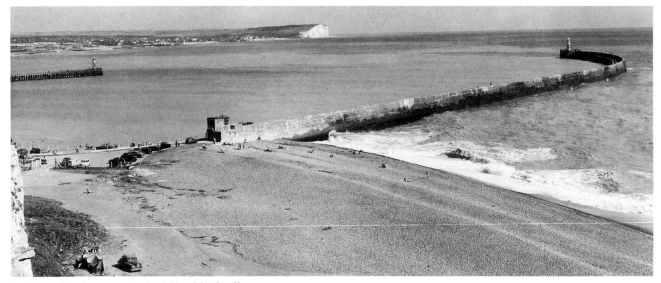

6.2 *Outer breakwaters. Seaford Head in the distance*

h. before HW. In the entrance it reaches 2 knots at Springs turning at approximately HW and LW.

Signals Harbour control is located inside the breakwater at the western entrance to the harbour itself. Traffic is controlled by signals as follows.

	By day	*By night*
Entry permitted	R triangle over R ball	G all-round
Departure permitted	R ball over R triangle	R all-round

	By day	*By night*
Free to move in or out	R ball	G Lt over R
No movement permitted .	R ball over R triangle over R ball	Lts RGR (Vert)

River Ouse Swing Bridge traffic signals:

Fl G	Bridge moving
Fl R	Ships may proceed downstream
FG	Ships may proceed upstream

Lights, etc. At end of outer (western) breakwater Oc (2) W 10s. 17m 12M dia ev 30s. in fog; at end of east pier, Iso G 5s. 12m 6M. Small F R Lt on W pier and F G on E pier, a cable inside entrance. Tide-gauge near base of lighthouse on W pier. When entering at night keep F R on Packet Wharf open between F R and F G Lts on W and E piers.

Radio D/F, call sign 'NH', on 303.4 kHz located at W entrance alongside traffic signals.

Anchorage and Berths

(1) *Outside off Seaford* in settled weather, but dangerous if wind shifts onshore.

(2) All yachts should seek instructions from Harbour Watch-house on W side of harbour (call on VHF Ch 16 or 12). Space is limited.

(3) Berthing and hauling out facilities are available in the *355- berth marina in Sleeper's Hole*, 3 cables within entrance on porthand side. Marine Watch-house at inshore end of southern marina jetty, or call on Ch 37 (Marina band), tel. 0273–513881.

Facilities Fuel and water from marina fuelling pontoon. Ship chandlers, and all stores obtainable. EC Wed. Yacht yard, yacht marina, gridirons and scrubbing hard. Launching site at Sleeper's Hole on application to marina office. Yacht club: Newhaven & Seaford SC. Station and numerous buses to all parts. Customs. A convenient port for those going to Glynde-bourne Opera.

Weather   BBC shipping forecast area: Wight.
Marinecall 0898–500456.
Radio Southern Sound 1323 kHz, on the hour and half hour.
BBC Radio Sussex on 1485, 1161 or 1368 kHz half-hourly 0630–0830, thence on the hour.
Hastings CG on Ch 7 at 0803–2003.

7 Brighton Marina

Charts: BA 1991; Im C9; Stan 9

High Water *as for Dover.*
Heights above Datum *MHWS 6m5. MLWS 0m7. MHWN 5m1. MLWN 1m9.*
Depths *Dredged to 2m5 at the entrance and 3m0 along the fairway inside shelving to 1m5 as on plan. The inner (non-tidal) basin is maintained at 2m4.*
Shoaling down to 1m0 at MLWS may occur off the end of the E breakwater, so favour the port hand once in the fairway.

THIS IMPRESSIVE artificial harbour, which has been built out into the Channel from Black Rock 1 mile east of the Palace Pier, Brighton, is the biggest marina development in Europe. It provides berths for 1,850 boats. About half the inner basin has been filled in to provide more housing, a superstore and leisure centre. It is an accessible port of refuge for yachts making the passage from the Straits of Dover to the Solent.

Approach and Entrance The marina is enclosed by a ¾ mile long eastern breakwater and a western one which extends farther to seaward to protect the entrance from W to SSW. In strong winds from the SE the outer entrance can be very rough, but the double entrance, spending beach and wave screen ensure that it is always calm inside. The recommended all-weather approach is to line up the Lt at the head of the W breakwater with the broad W stripe on the high-rise hospital building on the skyline on a course of 300° (see pic 7.2). In westerly winds do not shape to cut close round the W pierhead, since waves tend to bounce back there.

Lights At the end of the W breakwater there is a Lt Q R 9½m 7M. In fog there is a dia (2) ev 30s. Also at end of W bkwtr

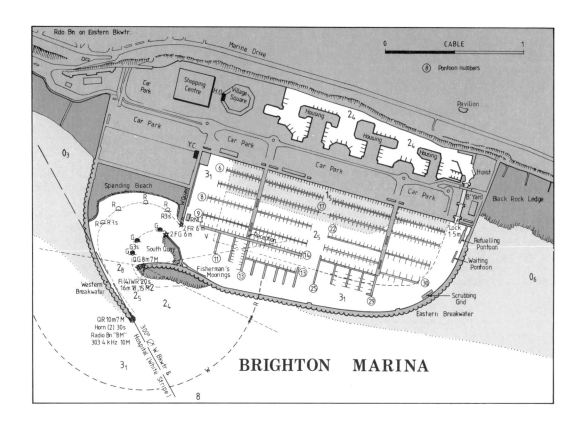

Rdo. Bn on Eastern Bkwtr.

Marine Drive

0   CABLE   1

⑧ Pontoon numbers

Car Park

Shopping Centre

H.O.

Village Square

Housing

Pavilion

2₄

Car Park

Car Park

2₄

Housing

Y.C.

Car Park

Housing

Hoist

0₃

⑥

3₁

B'Yard

Black Rock Ledge

Spending Beach

⑧

1₅

Car Park

R   R   R

R3s

⑰

Lock

1·5m

R   R3s

⑨

RNLI

R3s

2FR 6m

2FG 6m

South Quay

Refuelling Pontoon

G

⑪

Reception

2₅

㉒

⑭

Waiting Pontoon

G3s

V

G

IQG 8m7M

Fisherman's Moorings

⑬

⑬

⑤

0₆

2₈

Western Breakwater

Fl(4)WR 20s 16m 18,15 M2

⑤

㉕

3₁

㉚

Scrubbing Grid

2₅

⑤

㉙

2₄

Eastern Breakwater

QR 10m7M
Horn (2) 30s
Radio Bn "BM"
303·4 kHz 10M

300° Qc W Bkwtr &
Hospital (White Stripe)

W

R

BRIGHTON MARINA

3₁

8

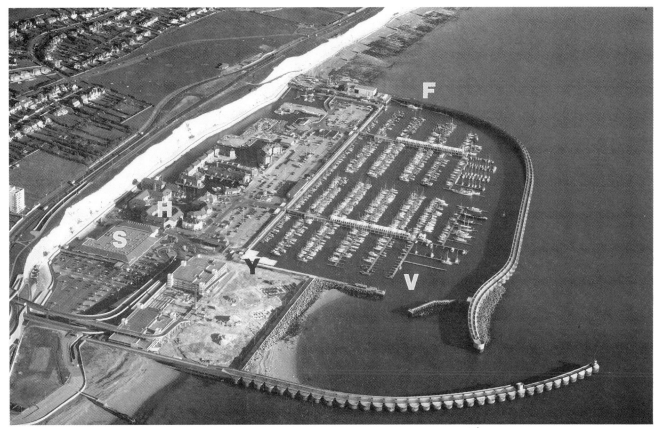

7.1 *Brighton Marina (1990). (H) Harbour Office (F) Fuel pontoon near lock to inner basin (Y) New Yacht Club (V) Visitor's berths (S) Supermarket*

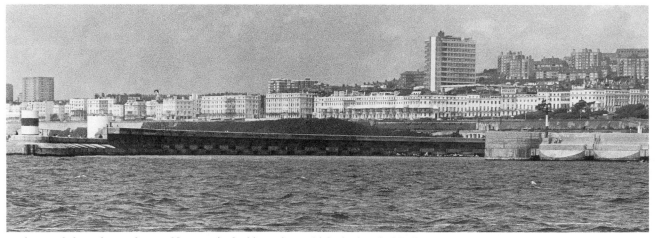

7.2 *Approach from the south-east. Note vertical white stripe on high-rise hospital building, rear transit for entry on 300°*

is a Rdo DF call-sign 'BM' on 303.4 kHz with range 10M. At the end of the E breakwater there is the principal lighthouse Fl (4) WR 20s. 16m 10M, with its R sector between 260° and 295°, white 295° through N to 100° and obscured elsewhere. At the same point is a Q G 8m 7M.

The entrance channel is marked by four R can buoys to port. Nos 2 and 6 have Fl R 3s., while the second of the three G con buoys to starboard has Fl G 3s. The inner pierheads are marked by 2 F R and 2 F G (Vert) to port and starboard respectively.

Harbour and Facilities   The layout of the berths is shown on the plan. In the tidal basin there are pontoon berths for boats up to 30m long with draughts ranging from 3m0 to 1m5. The HM will allocate berths on VHF Ch 37 or after the visitor has secured alongside the first pontoon on the porthand after entry.

The fuelling pontoon is at the NE corner near the lock-gates to the non-tidal basin, boatyard and travel-hoist. Inside the locked basin are berths for boats up to 18m long drawing 2m4. Priority is given to householders. Between the two harbours there are car parks, chandlery, and a massive shopping complex catering for all needs. The Brighton Marina YC welcomes visitors. A new clubhouse is being built in NW corner of Outer Harbour, tel. 0273–697049. There is a brokerage service and space for winter lay-up. In Brighton there are all the amenities of a large seaside town, with regular fast trains to London and others along the South Coast.

Weather   See Newhaven p. 69.
Brighton 0273–550266.

*8   Shoreham

Charts: BA 2044; Im C9; Stan 9

High Water *+ooh. 0.3m. Dover.*
Heights above Datum *at entrance MHWS 6m2. MLWS om7. MHWN 5mo. MLWN 1m9.*
Depths *The lowest charted depth in the approach is 1m7 LAT and 2m1 in the entrance. The dredged depths within the harbour are shown on the plan.*

SHOREHAM HARBOUR consists of a western arm which is the mouth of River Adur, and a short eastern arm leading through lock-gates to the Southwick Canal. Shoreham has few attractions for visiting yachtsmen unless a berth inside the locks is available, best by pre-arrangement after calling the HM on Ch 16 or 14 or by telephone on 0273–592613. There is a lot of commercial traffic (timber, coke, liquid gas and plonk in bulk) which takes priority through the locks or uses up most of the wharf frontage along the N bank of the River Adur.

It has, however, excellent communications by rail or bus to Brighton and London. It also has the distinction of being closer to an international airport than any other yacht harbour along the South Coast, with scheduled services to France and the Channel Islands, a flying school, aero club and readily available charter services. The ever-present dredger can be contacted on Ch 11.

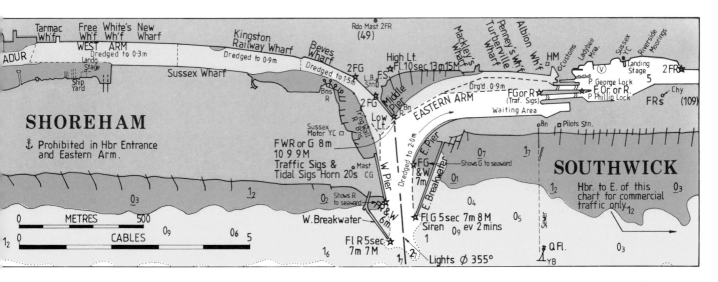

Approach and Entrance Shoreham harbour entrance is about 4 miles W of Brighton Palace Pier. The most conspicuous landmark is the chimney (marked at night by R Lts) of the power station about a mile ENE of the entrance. The entrance itself lies between two conspicuous concrete breakwaters. An unlit YB south cardinal buoy nearly 3 cables ESE of the entrance marks the outer end of a sewer outfall.

The shallowing water in the approach off the entrance can be very rough in strong onshore winds, particularly on the ebb tide. Newhaven or Brighton are better ports of refuge.

The entrance lies between the two concrete breakwaters within which are E and W piers. Farther north there is a third pier (the middle pier) on the fork of the western and eastern arms.

The leading lights consist of a lower light on the watch hut at the end of the middle pier and a higher one from a grey Lt Ho beyond. The structures are conspicuous by day, and approach to the harbour is best made on their transit at 355°. A radio mast (49) is just to the left of the transit.

Off the entrance the W-going stream starts about 2 h. before

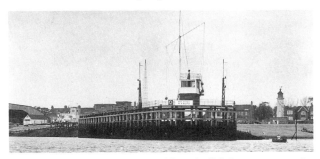

8.1 *Middle Pier watch-house, with main lighthouse open to the right and conspicuous TV mast to the left*

HW and the E-going 6 h. later. During the W-going stream there is a SW set across the entrance from the E breakwater towards the W breakwater, where part of it is deflected into the entrance and then NE towards the end of the E pier. The eddy is strongest 1 h. before HW to ebb 1 h. after HW.

The maximum rate of the main stream at the harbour entrance is about 3 knots, but the flood sets into the western arm, where it can attain 4 knots, and the ebb 5 knots in some parts at Springs. In the eastern arm there is practically no stream, but a yacht should be piloted with caution in the vicinity of the division off the middle pier.

The channel in the eastern arm is dredged and leads to the locks into the Southwick Canal. The western arm is only suitable for visiting yachts if able to take the ground. Traffic signals, given below, *must* be observed.

The locks are manned only 4 h. either side of HW and open about once an hour for traffic in each direction.

Traffic Control Signals All movements in the harbour and through the locks are controlled by International Port Movement light signals, shown from the watch-house on Middle Pier and at the locks. The addition of a Y light to any of the 3 Vert lights indicates that small craft need not comply, after receiving permission from Duty Control Officer.

Coastguards The prominent CG station just alongside the W side of the entrance is now in a care and maintenance state, only manned occasionally by volunteers. It is now part of the network controlled by Solent CG at Lee-on-Solent (tel. 0705–552100).

Lights E breakwater Lt Fl G 5s. 7m 8M. W breakwater Lt Fl R 5s. 7m 7M. These breakwater lights are not always easy to pick up against the background of bright lights. Leading lights (in transit 355° true). High Lt (rear) Fl W 10 s. 13m 15M. Low Lt (front) F W R or G (according to International Port Code) 8m. 10, 9, 9M. *Fog Signals.* E breakwater: siren ev 2m. Middle

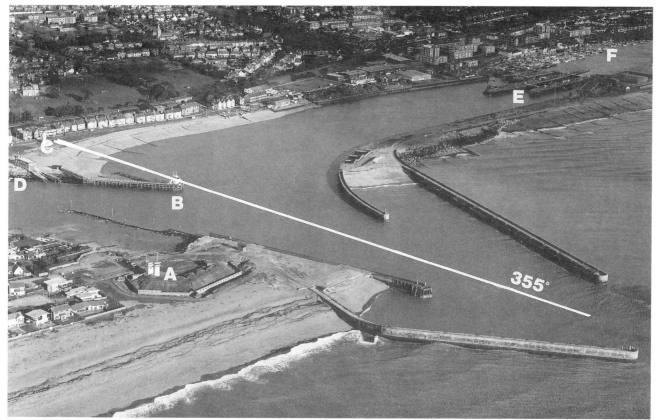

8.2 *(A) Coastguard (not manned) (B) Entry transit 355° of watch-tower and (C) Lighthouse (D) Lifeboat station (E) Locks (F) Marina*

pier: horn ev 20s. The latter is only sounded when ships are approaching.

Anchorages and Berths

(1) *Outside* clear of fairway in offshore winds and settled weather; the bottom is mostly sand over clay or chalk.

(2) Directions for berthing inside the harbour may be obtained from the duty officer on the middle pier at all times, but the Harbour Authority is virtually without berthing facilities of its own for yachts. Waiting for the locks: yachts are usually directed to secure temporarily to the N of the fairway.

Berthing arrangements must be made with a local yard or marina. All the available berths along the W arm (R. Adur) dry out and there are many houseboats already there. James Taylor, the Shoreham clubhouse of the Sussex YC or the Lighthouse Club might be able to help. Inside the locks all available pontoon berths – about 300 in all – are let to berth-holders, but call on Ch 37 or by tel. to the Lady Bee Marina on 0273-593801, or Riverside Marine on 07917-64831 or Surry Boatyard on 61491. The Southwick clubhouse of Sussex YC is near by. Yachts may not proceed E of this point without explicit permission of the HM, to whom you must report your arrival on the day of arrival. The HO and Customs House are both within a few minutes walk from any of these berths, tel. 0703–229251.

Facilities Water may be obtained at each marina. Fuel at the local garage near by. Full repair and chandlery services. There is a dry-dock and several slipways. Launching site from the beach next to the lighthouse and from several public hards. Car parking for any length of time is dodgy: best to make arrangements at one of several near-by garages.

Weather See Newhaven p. 69.

*9 Littlehampton

Charts: BA 1991; Im 9; Stan 9

High Water *at entrance* +00h. 0.4m. *Dover.*
Heights above Datum *MHWS* 5m7. *MLWS* 0m5.
MHWN 4m6. *MLWN* 1m7.
Depths *About 0m2 on bar, deepening between piers to about 1m2 to 2m4, which depths are maintained almost as far as the swingbridge.*

LITTLEHAMPTON at the mouth of the River Arun is a convenient harbour for yachts except for its bar (0m2 but subject to change) which can only be crossed with sufficient tide. Allowance has to be made for the strong streams in the entrance, and it is dangerous to approach in strong onshore winds. There is commercial shipping in the harbour but good facilities for yachts, with the town close by. Half a mile above the swingbridge a new bridge has been built, which has about 3m6 headroom at MHWS. The railway bridge at Ford has a clearance of 3m3 at HW. At Arundel a new road bridge has been built ¼ mile downstream of the old bridge with a clearance of 3m0 at MHWS. Craft which can pass under the bridges can navigate as far as Arundel, with a least depth of 1m3 MLWS the whole way.

Approach and Entrance The harbour is situated 10 miles E of Selsey Bill. Its entrance lies between two piers easily recognizable from seaward; 2½ miles to the SSW is the Winter Knoll YB south cardinal buoy (Q (6) + LFl 10s.). The western pier is the longer, and at its seaward end is a R Bn with a barrel top mark and Lt 2F R (Vert) 7m 6M.

The eastern pier stops short at the esplanade, but there is a low training wall for about ¼ mile seaward This is submerged from half tide to HW, but is marked by perches with X-topmarks and at its seaward end a G unlit Bn with W triangular topmark. The leading marks for the entrance on 346° are the W peppermill-shaped Lt Ho (Oc WY 7.5s 9m 10M) at the inshore end of the exposed E breakwater and the B steel column for the Lt (FG 6m 7M) at its seaward end in transit. Often the iron column may only be visible by day when it is in line with the W background of the Lt Ho. If the current is setting on to the W pier, keep nearer the eastern side. The tide is fierce in the narrow harbour entrance. Outside it turns to the W nearly 2 hours before HW. The approach should not be attempted in strong onshore winds and on the ebb tide the entrance can be very rough. Newhaven or Brighton are better ports of refuge. Speed limit 6.5 kts.

Signals When black-hulled pilot boat with large white 'P' at bow flies a R W flag by day, or shows W over R Lts by night, all boats keep clear, as a ship is about to enter or leave harbour. If ship signals one long and two short blasts, keep clear, particularly of narrows at entrance.

Anchorage

(1) *Outside*, S of entrance at distance according to vessel's draught: this is slightly sheltered from the W by Selsey Bill and the Owers but is completely open from the SW, through S to ENE.

(2) Visiting yachts may secure temporarily *alongside County Wharf* on the E bank immediately above the ferry (which has right of way at all times). The HM whose office is on this wharf will then direct visitors to a berth, if one is available. Do NOT anchor in the fairway or secure to a pontoon berth on the west bank – they are privately owned, 100 of them by the Arun YC. The HM can be contacted by telephone on 0903–721215/6. Arun YC on 0903–714553.

(3) There are 120 afloat berths for boats drawing up to 2m1 – some always kept for visitors – at the Littlehampton marina on

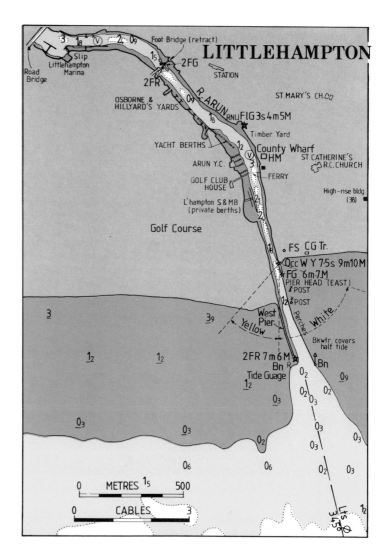

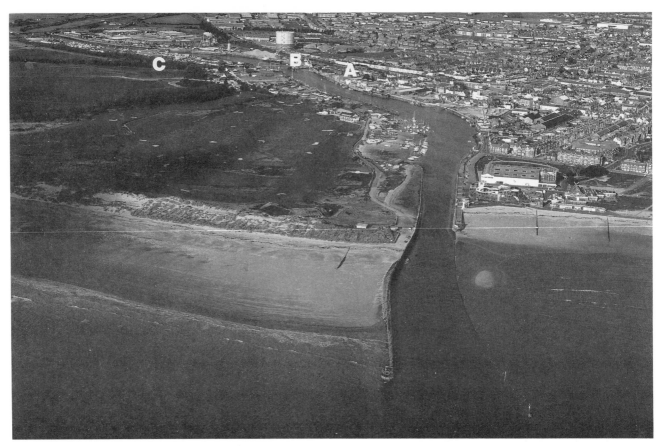

9.1 *(A) Harbour Master (B) Footbridge (C) Littlehampton Marina*

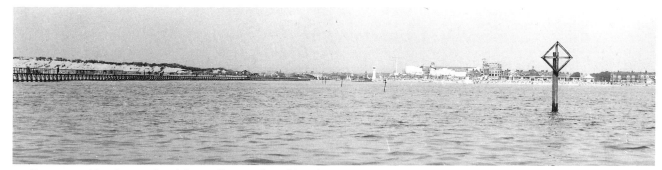

9.2 *Entrance with submerged training wall on starboard hand*

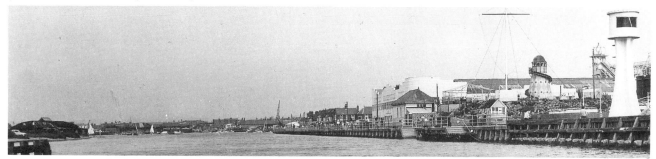

9.3 *Unusual lighthouse on the east bank near entrance*

the left bank upstream from the retractable footbridge, clearance 1m8 at MHWS. River traffic controlled by lights: R indicates channel closed, G means it is open. Contact on Ch 37 or 0903–713553.

Facilities Water, fuel and repairs at any of the four boatyards on the river or at the marina, which also has a slip, lift and chandlery. All shopping in the town. Yacht clubs: Arun YC, Littlehampton S & MB. Good connections by rail or bus.

Weather BBC shipping forecast area: Wight.
See Newhaven p. 69.

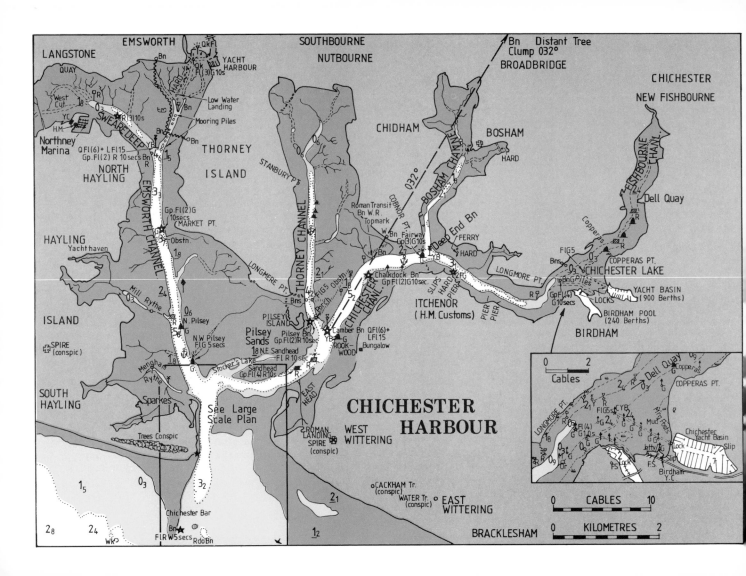

CHICHESTER HARBOUR

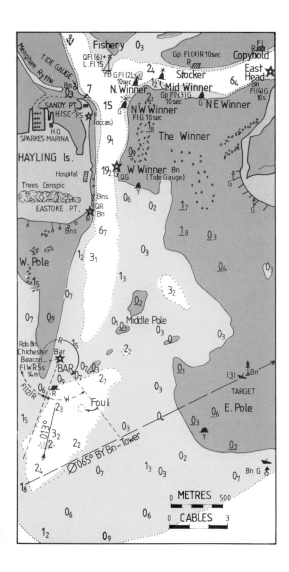

*10   Chichester Harbour

Charts: BA 3418; Im Y33; Stan 10

High Water *at entrance +00h. 11m. Dover.*

Heights above Datum   *MHWS 4m9. MLWS 0m7. MHWN 4m0. MLWN 1m8.*

Depths   *The water starts to shoal nearly a mile south of the Chichester Bar Bn. On the correct approach the least water on the bar is dredged to 2m0 at MLWS, but less than a cable either side it dries. After severe gales it can vary ±0m75. The entrance between the E end of Hayling Island and the Winner Sands is deep (as much as 19m). Except for a patch (1m4) just NE of the N Winner buoy, the main fairway has not less than 2m4 as far as Itchenor in one direction and the Emsworth S cardinal buoy in the other.*

CHICHESTER HARBOUR is an ideal small boat centre, with over 17 miles of navigable water within its sheltered limits. There is racing for all small classes, so it is hardly surprising that there are 14 sailing clubs here, more than in any other S Coast harbour. No less than 10,000 boats over 3m long are based here, 2,000 of them alongside in five marinas. Bosham, Emsworth, Itchenor and Birdham are all attractive villages well worth visiting. There is an 8-knot speed limit throughout the harbour.

The whole area is controlled by the Chichester Harbour Conservancy through the Manager/HM at Itchenor, tel. 0243–512301 or using call-sign 'CHICHESTER' on Ch 16 or 14 on which VHF watch is kept 0900–1730. He can advise on berthing availability anywhere in the whole harbour. His launch is *Regnum*.

Approach and Entrance   The entrance to Chichester harbour lies some 8 miles west of Selsey Bill. There are

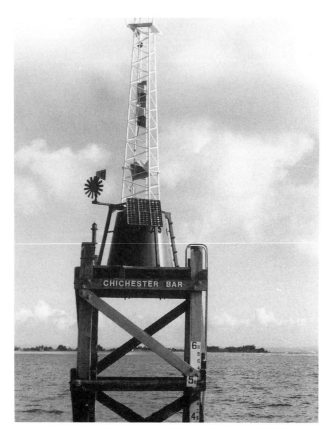

10.1 *Chichester Bar Beacon showing 3m5 on tide gauge, with Sandy Point open to the right (John Crampton)*

extensive sands extending seaward on both sides of the approach and entrance, named the West Pole, the Middle Pole and the East Pole. With strong onshore winds there can be a very ugly sea on the bar, especially on the ebb running 6½ knots at Springs when the approach can be dangerous. At Springs or in rough weather it is advisable to cross the bar 3 h. before HW to 1 h. after.

When approaching from E or W keep well offshore outside 5mo line until one or both of the conspicuous marks have been identified – the Nab Tr bearing 184° or Chichester Bar Bn (Fl W R 5s. 14m) bearing 004°. It has a Ro Bn call-sign 'CH' range 10M with coded wind information. Long dashes (1–8 clockwise starting at 1 for NE) and one short dot for each Beaufort wind Force. Frequency 303.4 kHz.

Coming from the westward, get on the transit of the stranded target on E Pole Sands, marked by a N-cardinal Bn and the Cakeham Tower in the Witterings on course 064°. Then alter course for the Bar Bn, which should be left close to port. The water shoals rapidly from 1 mile S of the Bn to 2mo at the Bn, where there is a tide-gauge which gives the level at chart datum. The principal dangers are the E Pole sands, which extend over a mile SE of the Bn, and the spit of the W Pole now running nearly 2 cables to seaward of the Bn. This is covered by a narrow Fl R (2) 10s. sector from the Bn and, in summer by an R con buoy to seaward of the Bar.

When Chichester Bar is abeam, the entrance to Chichester harbour lies immediately E of Eastoke Point, just clear of the right-hand edge of the trees on the sandy point. The distance from ½ cable E of the Chichester Bar Bn to the entrance is about a mile making good a course of 013° on the West Winner Bn (Q G) which has tide gauges on it. This course has been dredged to 1m5 below CD, keeping clear of the W Pole and Middle Pole Sands.

The water soon becomes much deeper. Leave Eastoke Bn

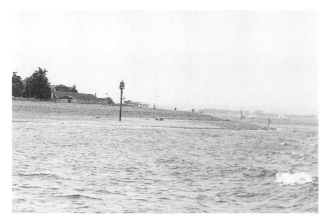

10.2 *Eaststoke Beacon marking porthand limit of entrance with dangerous eddy 50m to its east. Conspicuous hospital buildings demolished as part of redevelopment.*

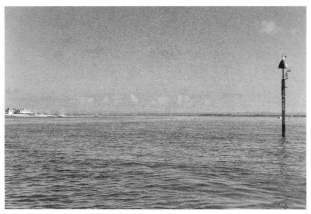

10.3 *West Winner Beacon to starboard, with Hayling Island Sailing Club on the left (John Crampton)*

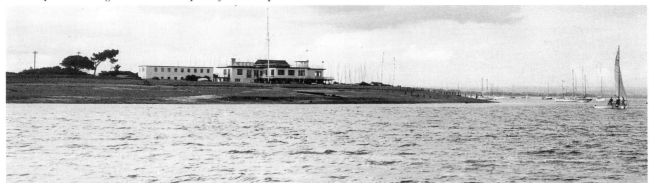

10.4 *Hayling Island Sailing Club and Sandy Point, beyond which the channel to Sparkes' Marina leads westwards*

83

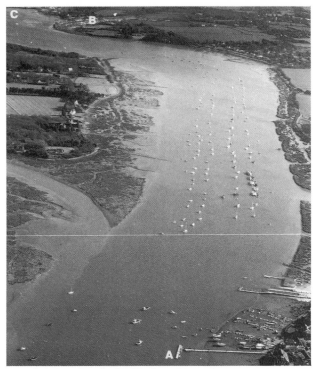

10.5 *Itchenor Reach. (A) Harbour Master's pontoon (B) Birdham Pool (C) Chichester Yacht Basin*

(Q R) and small unlit Bns at the ends of groynes to port and alter to follow the entrance channel between the steep shingle shore on the port hand and the wide expanse of the Winner sands on the starboard hand. These dry at LW and are marked by the W Winner Bn and the N-W Winner buoy (G 10s.). In the entrance channel the tidal streams are fierce and may attain 2.8 knots on the flood or 6.4 knots on a big Spring ebb about 2 h. after HW.

Within the entrance the channel divides into two arms. One leads in a northerly direction to Emsworth and is entered between Sandy Point with Hayling Is SC prominent and the S-cardinal Fishery buoy (Q (6) + Fl 15s.). It is wide and deep nearly as far as the junction with Sweare Deep, where there is the YB south cardinal Emsworth Bn (Q (6) + L Fl 15s.). Another 0.8 miles on a NW'ly course the Sweare Deep R Bn (Fl (3) R 10s.) off the R Northney Bn (Fl (4) R 10s.) is the entrance to the Northney Marina on the N tip of Hayling Island and beyond it the narrow W Cuts channel leading under Langstone bridge – strictly for boats of less than 8ft superstructure above their waterline, and at the right tide.

The other channel from the Emsworth Bn is the mile-long front drive to the Emsworth Yacht Harbour. This channel dries for most of its length beyond the R Fisherman's Bn (Fl (3) R 10s.)

From the Fishery buoy the other arm bears round the N side of the Winner to the eastward and leads via the Chichester Channel to Itchenor, the Bosham Channel and to Dell Quay.

To enter the Chichester Channel (after passing Hayling Is SC and Sandy Point on the W side) bear to starboard to the eastward to leave to starboard the NW Winner (Fl G 10s.), the G conical N Winner (Fl (2) G 10s.), the Mid Winner (Gp Fl (3) 10s.) conical buoys and the East Head Bn (Fl (4) G 10s.) with tide-gauge. There is a shoal patch 1m5 close NNE of the N Winner buoy but otherwise the channel is from 2m4 to 7m deep. Leave to port the following R can buoys: Stocker (Gp Fl (3) R 10s.), Copyhold (unlit) and Sandhead (Fl (4) R 10s.).

The next pair of buoys are the NE Sandhead (Fl R 10s.) to port and the G Rookwood buoy to starboard. East of the NE Sandhead buoy the channel bears to the NE, where identify and bring Roman Transit Bn (R porthand daymark) in transit with the main channel Bn (white rectangular daymark) on the shore at 032° with Stoke Clump, a conspicuous clump of trees on the distant downs. If it is too misty to see these landmarks it does not matter, for the channel is clearly marked on the port hand by the YB S-cardinal Camber Bn (Q (6) + LFl 15s.) at the entrance of the Thorney Channel and on the starboard hand by the Chalkdock Bn (Fl (2) G 10s.) and by occasional perches, though these are situated high up on the mud and should be given a wide berth near low water.

After passing the Chalkdock Bn alter course to round the G conical starboard-hand Fairway buoy (Gp Fl (3) G 10s.) at the junction of the Bosham and Chichester Channels. Close to the NE is the Deep End YB south cardinal Bn which is an unlit starboard-hand mark for the Bosham Channel and a port-hand one for the Itchenor Reach. This channel is deep almost as far as Longmore Point about a mile east of Itchenor, where it then shallows but is marked by buoys. Access to Dell Quay and the Chichester Yacht Basin needs help from the tide.

The Bosham Channel carries 1m8 to within 2 cables of the quay at the village and is marked by R and G perches.

The Thorney Channel is entered by leaving the S-cardinal Camber Bn (Q Fl (6) + Fl 15s.) to starboard, and then leaving Pilsey Island R Bn (Fl (2) R 10s.) to port and a G perch to starboard; neither should be passed close to. Then pass between a pair of Bns beyond which the channel is straight and marked by R and G perches. Depths range from 3m7 down to 1m8 to NE of Stanbury Point.

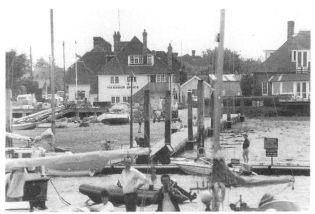

10.6 *Harbour Master's pontoon at Itchenor*

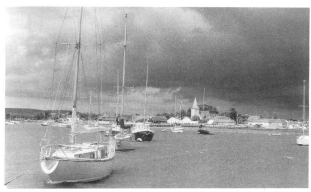

10.7 *Moorings in Bosham channel, with Old Bosham Church in background*

Anchorages and Berthing

(1) In westerly winds just within the entrance north of *Sandy Point* outside local moorings.

(2) *Off East Head*, beyond the Bn. Pleasant anchorage on sandy bottom in settled weather, but very crowded in summer and rather exposed except from S and E. A shallow creek marked by perches leads to the Roman Landing and West Wittering SC.

(3) *In Chichester Channel* on the south of the channel leading to the Fairway buoy.

(4) At *Itchenor* visiting yachts up to 10 tons should moor temporarily at one of six visitors' buoys (W with R band), each taking six boats abreast, opposite the HM's office. Contact on VHF Ch 16 or 14 or telephone (0243–512301). The HM or his deputy will then allocate a vacant mooring of which some are usually available.

(5) *In the marinas at Birdham Pool or the Chichester Yacht Basin*. Allow for sufficient tide as the main channel dries out at MLWS soon after passing Longmore Point. The 250-berth Birdham Pool is normally accessible at half tide. To reach it, leave the G Birdham Bn (Gp Fl (4) G 10s.) to port and the line of unlit perches leading to the lock-gates close to starboard, disregarding another line farther off the retaining wall, since they point the way to the Birdham YC slip. To reach the 1000-berth Chichester Yacht Basin, continue up channel from the Birdham Bn for a further 2 cables to the G Yacht Basin Bn (Fl G 5 sec.), then leave close to starboard the six G piles leading to the lock. This channel is dredged to 1m1. Depths inside both these marinas may vary from time to time, so yachts drawing 2m0 or more must seek directions for berthing at the lock-gates. Both marinas have all the facilities expected of a major yacht harbour.

(6) *Bosham Lake*. This historic village is charming, but the creek is full of private moorings and it dries out within 2 cables of the quay. Apply locally or to the HM at Itchenor for temporary facilities or to dry out alongside. There is a public slip on which to leave a dinghy.

(7) *Thorney Channel* provides a well-protected anchorage where space can be found. Facilities ashore are limited to those provided by the Thorney Island SC. The island is under Ministry of Defence control, so that permission must be obtained at the guardroom for access by road. A few drying berths are available on pontoons at Andrews Yacht Harbour at Thornham off the Prinstead Channel, tel. 0243–375335.

(8) *The Emsworth Channel* is suitable for anchoring almost anywhere on the E side as far as its junction with Sweare Deep, but keep clear of the W side due to private moorings and Fishery Orders. The HM added 90 extra moorings in this reach during 1987 so may well have a spare. Beyond the YB S-cardinal Emsworth Bn (Q (6) + LFl ev 15s.) there are pile moorings in trots on the port hand for shoal draught boats. At the NE end of the channel is the Emsworth Yacht Harbour (220 berths). It is advisable to call 0243–43065 to check availability and depths at the entrance, which vary between 2m7 at Spring and 2m5 at Neaps.

(9) *The Northney Marina* at the northern end of Hayling Island just short of the Langstone Bridge has 260 berths for boats drawing 1m8 (tel. 0705–466321). It has excellent facilities, backed by a modern conference hotel and its own residential clubhouse.

(10) *Sparkes Yacht Harbour* with 140 pontoon berths and all the facilities of an active yacht yard lies immediately W of Sandy Point, the home of the Hayling Island SC, at the end of its own 2m0 dredged channel. Berths have depths up to 2m2 afloat at MLWS. One of its attractions is that it is only 1½ miles from Chichester Bar. Contact on Ch 37 or by tel. 0705–463572.

Facilities At Itchenor there are yacht yards and marine engineers. Landing and water by hose at the floating jetty, where there is a tide-gauge. H. C. Darnley & Sons supply chandlery and will fill petrol cans. No shops. The Ship Inn has

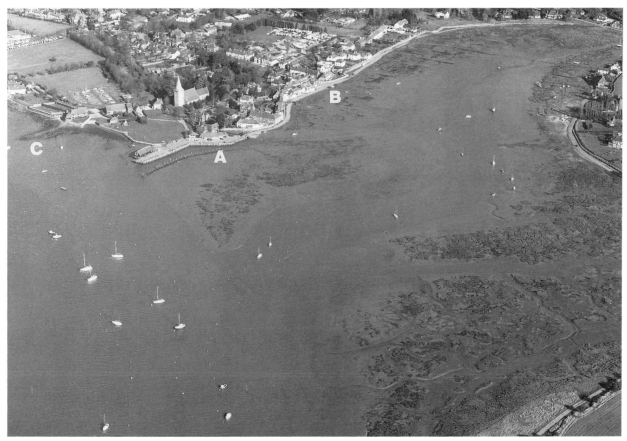

10.8 *Bosham reach. (A) Yacht Club (B) Public slip (C) Yacht Club slip*

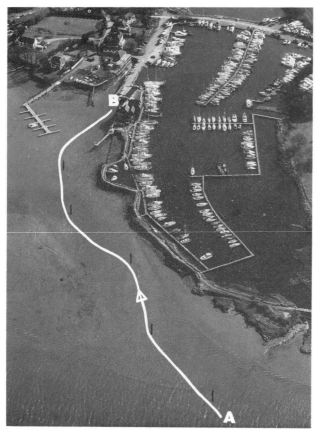

10.9 *Birdham Pool. Channel marked A–B to lock-gates,
leaving each beacon close to starboard*

six bedrooms and a restaurant; some provisions for visitors are available in summer. All facilities from both marinas at Birdham. Occasional buses to Chichester. At Bosham, yacht yards and sailmaker, PO and shops. EC Thurs. Buses to Chichester and Portsmouth. In the Emsworth Channel, yacht yards at Mengham Rythe and Mill Rythe. Emsworth itself is a small town where there is the yacht harbour and all facilities. Northney Marina and Sparkes Yacht Harbour provide all that a visiting yacht could require. EC Wed. Station and buses. Customs from Portsmouth (tel. Freephone Customs Yachts or tel. 0705–826511) but in the summer may often be close at hand. Their launch is berthed at Northney Marina.

Launching sites: (1) from public hards at end of roads at Itchenor, Bosham, Dell Quay, Thornham and Emsworth, with car parks near by. (2) Near HW at the NE side of Hayling Bridge at the slipway administered by the Langstone SC and also at Birdham YC and Dell Quay. (3) at Sandy Point by permission from the Hayling Island SC. (4) At Emsworth from public hard or Emsworth Yacht Harbour. Yacht clubs: Birdham YC, Bosham SC, Chichester Cruising Club (Itchenor), Chichester YC (Birdham), Dell Quay SC, Emsworth SC, Hayling Island SC, Itchenor SC, Langstone SC, Mengham Rythe SC, West Wittering SC, Thorney Island SC.

The *Chichester Harbour Guide* (£1.00) is informative and lucid.

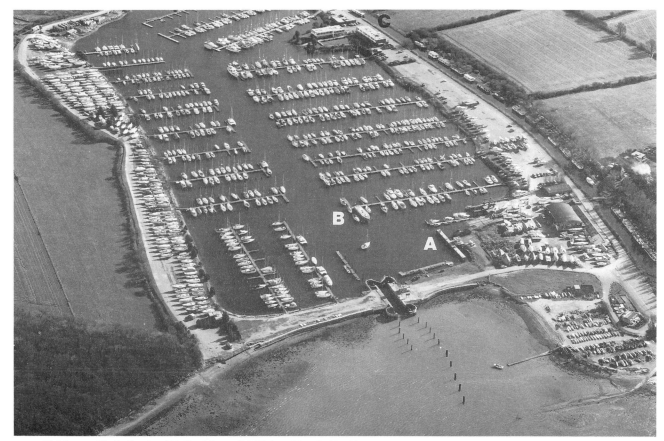

10.10 *Chichester Yacht Basin. (A) Fuel jetty (B) Visitors' berth (C) Chandlery and offices*

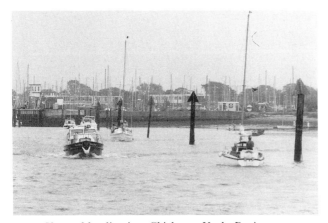

10.11 *Channel leading into Chichester Yacht Basin*

Weather BBC shipping forecast area: Wight.
Marinecall 0898–500457.
BBC Radio Solent on 300 and 221m (999 and 1359kHz) or 96.1MHz at 0633, 0745.
Ocean Sound East on 257m (1170kHz) or 97.5MHz at 0629, 0729, 0829, 1629, 1729 (not weekends).
By phone from Weathercall (Poole–Chichester) 0898–500403.
Niton Radio on Ch 28 (1834kHz) at 0833, 2033.
By phone from CG MRSC at Lee-on-Solent on 0705–552100. They guard Ch 16 and 2182kHz.

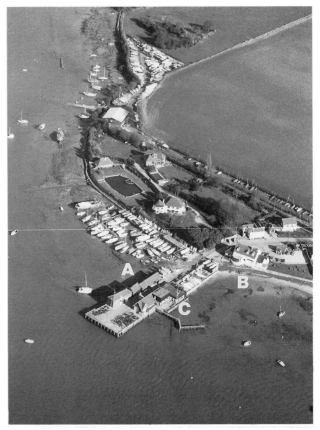

10.12 *Dell Quay. (A) Public slip (B) Pub (C) Dell Quay Yacht Club*

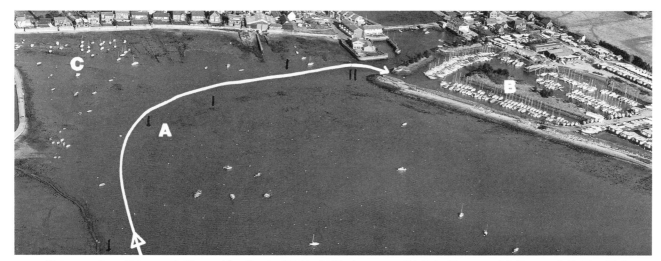

10.13 *Upper reaches of Emsworth Channel leading to (B) Yacht Harbour past (A) Echo Beacon, with Emsworth Sailing Club channel at (C)*

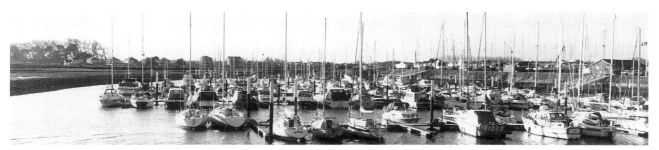

10.14 *Northney Marine from its entrance. Secure to nearest free pontoon*

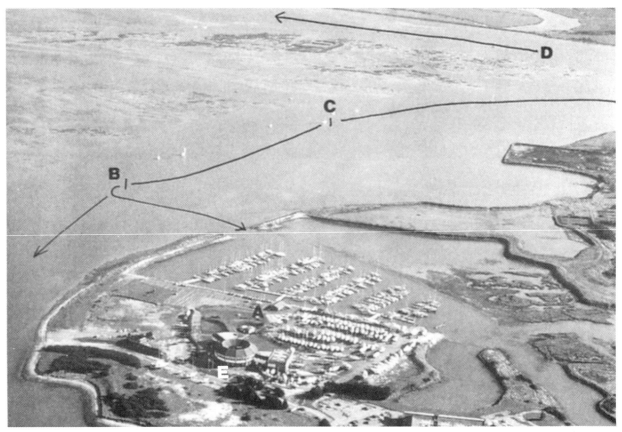

10.15 *Northney Marina. Approach past Sweare Deep beacon (C) and Northney beacon (B). (A) Harbour Office (E) Hotel (D) Emsworth Channel*

11 Langstone Harbour

Charts: BA 3428; Im Y33; Stan 10

High Water   +00h. 14m. Dover.
Heights above Datum *at entrance approx: MHWS 4m8.
MLWS 0m6. MHWN 3m9. MLWN 1m8.*
Depths   *The entrance varies, but there is not less tham 2m0
except over the bar between the E and W Winner sands. Within
the harbour over 2m in main channels.*

LANGSTONE HARBOUR is a fine area especially for centreboard
boats. There is also plenty of water for cruising yachts in the
main channels. Approach to Langstone Marina 0m6 above CD
allows 1m5 keels at LW.

Approach and Entrance   The entrance to Langstone
Harbour may be located by the high chimney on its west side,
but the channel leading to it lies between the extensive W and E
Winner sands. The RW Fairway buoy (Fl 10s.) is situated about
a mile offshore on Langstone Bar. The shoals and sands are
liable to change. Approach from the west may be made either
from the direction of the Horse Sand Fort or through the gap in
the submerged barrier a mile north of the fort. In either case
bring the Horse Sand Fort into line with the No Man's Land
Fort on a stern transit of 235° which leads to the isolated danger
BRB Roway wreck Bn (Fl (2) 5s.) SSW of the entrance. Least
water on this course is 1m8 between BRB Bn and the Langstone
Fairway buoy.

If taking the short cut from the Portsmouth direction pass
through the gap in the submerged barrier. The gap lies nearly a
mile S of Lumps Fort on the Eastney shore and is marked by a
dolphin Q R on the south side. Keep close to the dolphin in 1m2
as there is an obstruction on the NNW side. Then make good a

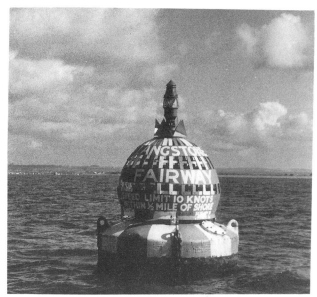

11.1 *Langstone Fairway buoy*

course of 090° until picking up the back transit of the big forts on
235°.

If approaching from the eastward the danger lies in the E
Winner sand, which dries out nearly ½ mile SE of the Fairway
buoy, and has an extension of shoal water with only 0m4 even a
mile SE of the Fairway buoy. The YB S-cardinal E Winner buoy
is about 4 cables south of the shoal. The buoy should be left to
northward and the course should not be altered until the
Fairway buoy bears N true which just clears the edge of the E

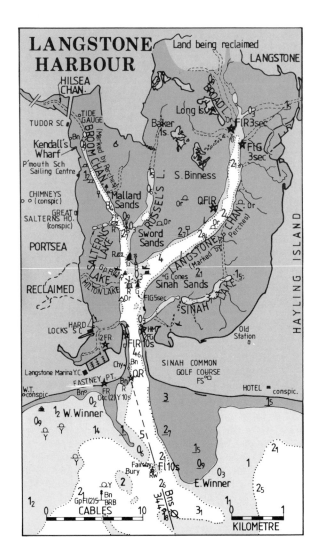

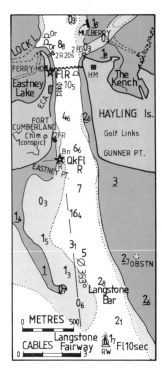

Winner shoal (1m8). Under reasonable conditions Langstone is an easy harbour to enter but the approaches can be dangerous in strong onshore winds, especially near LW on the ebb; the roughest part of all in southerly winds lies about a cable NNE of the Fairway buoy, 2 h. after HW when the ebb is at its maximum rate.

From the Fairway buoy initially make good a course of 353°

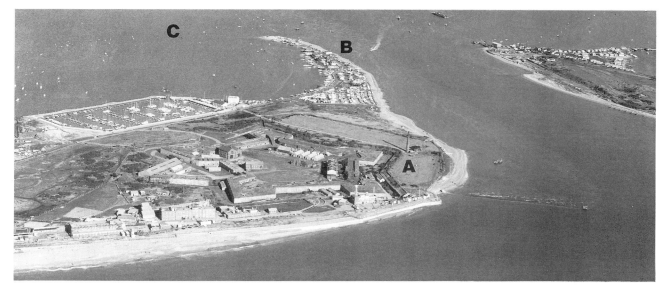

11.2 *(C) Entrance to marina by way of Lock's Lake (A) Conspicuous chimney (B) Yacht Club with Eastney Marina centre left*

towards the narrow entrance, favouring the W side of the channel. You are straying into danger if you get to the left of the 353° transit of the R Bn (Q R) at the seaward end of the first outfall and the rt-hand edge of land. A cable beyond the first R Bn there is a new pier with 2F R at its extremity. The tide often exceeds 3 kts in the bottleneck. Speed limit is 10 kts.

At the northern end of the entrance there is a R Bn (R 10s.) close to the Eastney Cruising Assn clubhouse, then two Fl R 20s. on the Eastney ferry pontoon. On the opposite side there are 2F G lts on the Hayling Island ferry pontoon. Thereafter navigate as desired to your chosen anchorage.

With the tide right, small craft without masts stepped can pass under Hayling roadbridge (2m1 clearance at MHWS) to the upper reaches of Chichester Harbour.

Anchorage and Facilities

(1) There are four round W visitors' buoys for temporary use *on the E side of the entrance* near the northern end and just S of the cable Bns. These are adjacent to the HM's office on Hayling Is.

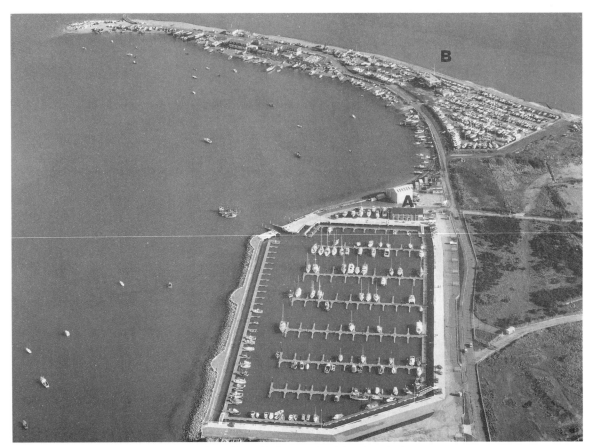

11.3 *Marina in Eastney Lake. (A) Marina office (B) Eastney Cruising Association*

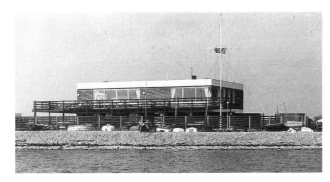

11.4 *Eastney Cruising Association clubhouse on west side*

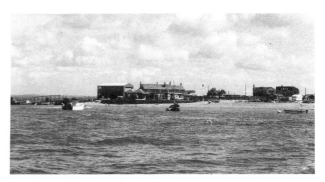

11.5 *East side of entrance*

Seek his advice for vacant moorings (tel. 0705–463419) or on Ch 16 or 12 during office hours. Close by there is a water point for filling cans. There is a boatyard where petrol or diesel fuel can be obtained or direct by dinghy about 1½ h. either side of HW. Other facilities are the Ferry Boat Inn, a café and general store. Launching site at slip. Bus service to Hayling village (EC Wed.) and Havant. Frequent ferries to Eastney in summer, thence bus to Portsmouth.

(2) *The Eastney Cruising Association* on W side of entrance (see harbour plan) has two fair-weather visitors' moorings (fierce tide for about 1 h. about 2 h. after HW); riding light necessary at night. The club is a do-it-yourself concern and hospitable; bar and meals in sailing season. Public launching site at end of road near ferry pontoon. Buses to Portsmouth in summer.

(3) *Langstone Marina* in Eastney Lake has 330 berths for boats drawing up to 2m4; 30 are reserved for visitors. Immediately N of sandy spit of land to port, the channel 0m6 above CD leads WSW between Bns with R and G topmarks. After 2 cables the channel swings to port directly for the marina entrance. Waiting pontoon just outside the entrance and sill has 1m7 below CD. It is normally open 14h. a day. Wait for R Lt on the port side of the entrance to turn G before entry. Boat-hoist, winter storage. Fuel and shore power. Tel. 0705–822719.

(4) *Eastney Lake* dries out and is full of moorings for small craft which take the mud at LW. The Lock SC has a clubhouse and concrete slip, with a general store near by.

(5) *Anywhere* that can be found on the edges of the main channel out of the fairway (which is used by ballast dredgers) and clear of moorings.

(6) *Langstone Channel*, although far from facilities, provides plenty of room to anchor in depths ranging from 5mo to 2mo E of South Binness Island. Launching sites from the foreshore at the end of the roads leading to the ferry on either side of the entrance, preferably at slack water as the tides run very hard. Car parks adjacent. Other YC: Tudor SC on W of Broom Channel.

Weather See Chichester p. 90.
Southampton Weather Centre 0703–228844.

12 Portsmouth Harbour

Charts: BA 2625, 2631; Im C3, C9; Stan 11

High Water +ooh. *14m. Dover.*
Heights above Datum *MHWS 4m7. MLWS om6. MHWN 3m8. MLWN 1m8. Flood 7 h. Ebb 5h.*
Depths *The entrance and main harbour are a deep ship channel. The Fareham Channel has 7 to 9m at the entrance, gradually shallows, and there is little water off Fareham;*

Portchester Channel is also deep as far as junction with Tipner Lake, but there is a dredged channel 1m5 below CD from the vicinity of Nos 72 and 77 Bns opposite Portchester Castle to the lock-gates at Port Solent.

PORTSMOUTH is indelibly linked with the Royal Navy's past and, to a lesser extent, its future. Nelson's flagship *Victory* towers over the Royal Dockyard, looking across the harbour towards the Submarine Museum up Haslar Creek with HMS *Alliance* parked above the tide. Either side of *Victory* are the reconstructed fragments of Henry VIII's *Mary Rose* and HMS

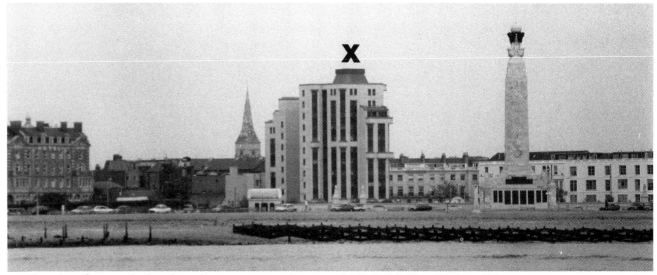

12.1 *Transit 048° across the Swashway here seen open to the west, with St Jude's Church spire still in view*

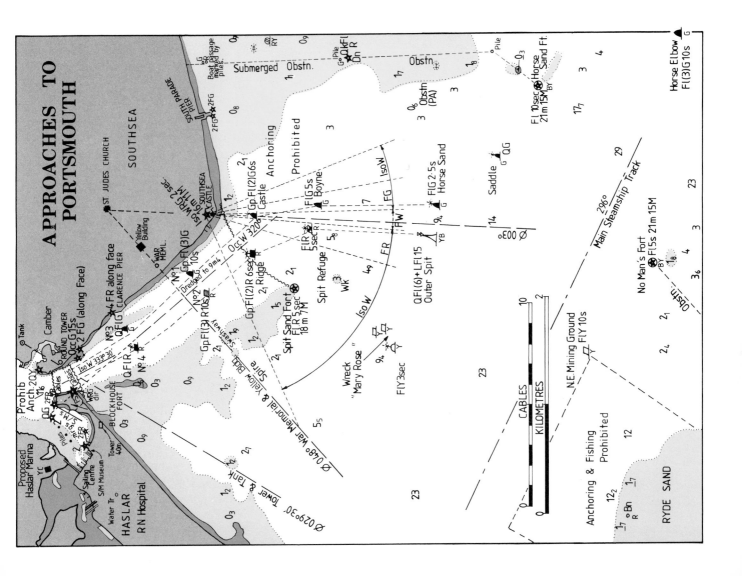

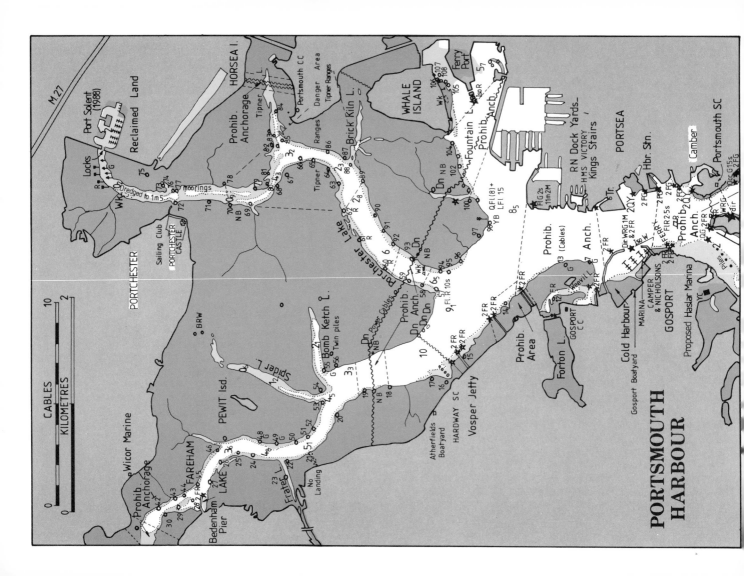

PORTSMOUTH HARBOUR

Warrior, recently restored from a hulk to be preserved as the first armoured battleship propelled by sail and steam. HM ships come and go, or stay for long refits. But the town's economy has been boosted by winning the cross-Channel ferry traffic from Southampton, now operating from a new terminal in Fountain Lake right off the the M27 spur. For yachtsmen Portsmouth is a safe and convenient port accessible at all states of the tide. Apart from several small piers mostly for Service use, there is a 350-

berth marina on the Gosport side (Camper & Nicholson's) backed by good boat-building and repair facilities. At the head of the shallow creek leading to Portchester there is a new 850-berth marina, Port Solent, for boats up to 42m LOA drawing 3m0. It is accessible at all states of the tide for boats drawing 1m5. The upper reaches and channels provide good small boat sailing. There is a speed limit of 10 knots within 900m of the shore in any part of the dockyard port. Water ski-ing is not permitted within the harbour. Boats with engines must use them from the Southsea War Memorial until clear inside the harbour, having followed the small craft channel on the Blockhouse side.

Approach and Entrance   From the eastward the approach is simple, being buoyed for big ships from the YB S-cardinal Outer Spit buoy (Q Fl (6) + L Fl 15s.) inward, as shown on the chart. From the westward leave Gilkicker Pt (Oc 6 10s. 7m) a cable to port, then pass 2 cables S of Spit Sand Fort (R 5s.), where course can be altered direct to the deep channel inshore of the Outer Spit buoy. A short cut across the Spit Sand giving 1m8 at MLWS ½ mile W of the Spit Sand Fort is by bringing into transit on 048° the War Memorial on Southsea front with a tall yellow building. Another swashway available (with sufficient tide above 0m3 at LAT) lies across the Hamilton Bank by

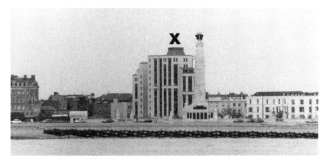

12.2 *Transit of War Memorial and brown top to yellow apartment building (X) nearly on*

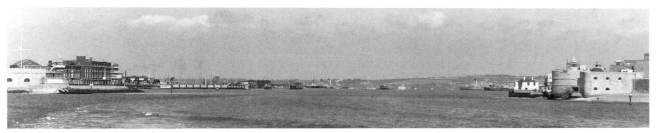

12.3 *Entrance between Fort Blockhouse on the left and Old Portsmouth on the right*

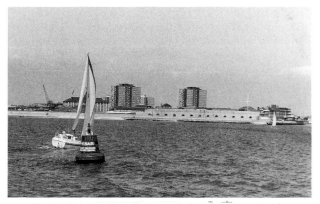

12.4 *Boat using small craft channel, leaving No. 4 bar buoy to starboard heading to pass close to Fort Blockhouse*

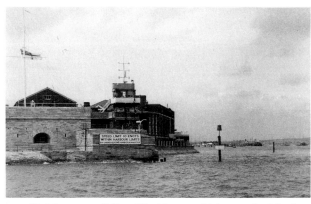

12.5 *Red beacons off Fort Blockhouse which must be left close outside by small craft*

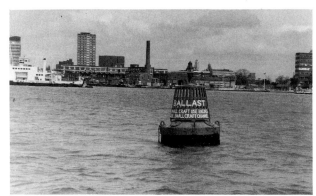

12.6 *Ballast Patch buoy off entrance to Haslar Creek. Small craft must pass to the west of it*

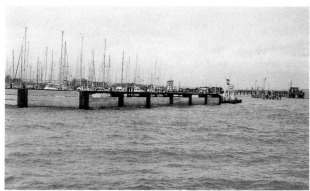

12.7 *Approach to Camper & Nicholson's Marina, with fuel barge at the end of wave baffle*

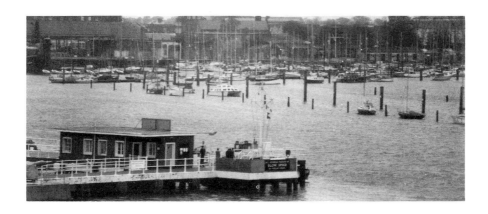

12.8 *Haslar Creek. HMS Dolphin pier with pile moorings opposite. Note HMS 'Alliance' top left, part of the Submarine Museum*

keeping the western edge of the Round Tr on the Portsmouth side of the harbour entrance in line with the left-hand edge of a conspicuous tank at 029½°. Daytime only.

The main big ship channel parallel to Southsea Common is marked at night by being within the 320° Oc W sector of the directional WRG Lt on Fort Blockhouse. If you are in the Oc G sector you are out of the channel to the N and should move over to the other side (Oc R) before you reach the No. 4 buoy (Q R), which yachts must leave to starboard, marking the seaward end of the Boat Channel. From here shape to pass as close as you dare to the unlit R Bns on the Blockhouse side of the channel and hold on to leave Ballast buoy (Fl R 2.5s.) on your starboard hand. In transiting the Boat Channel you should be in the Iso R 2s. sector of the directional Harbour Entrance Lt situated in the entrance to the Gosport (Camper's) marina on a course around 340°.

In the entrance itself the tides are very strong. The flood runs easy for 3 h., strong for 4 h.; the ebb easy 1 h., strong for from 2 to 3 h., and then easy. Maximum 3½ knots on flood, 5 knots on ebb.

Vessels approaching inshore from the eastward may pass through the gap in the submerged barrier. The gap is about a mile south of Lumps Fort and is marked by a dolphin (Q R) on the south. Many of the piles on the barrier have been removed, but the remains and many submerged concrete blocks still constitute a danger.

Haslar Creek running SW from Fort Blockhouse near the harbour entrance is full of private moorings and pontoon berths at the Joint Services Sail Training Centre just upstream from the Submarine Memorial (HMS *Alliance*). A new marina is proposed on its N side. Date uncertain.

Fareham Lake About 1½ miles from the entrance, Portsmouth harbour divides into two channels. The westward of the

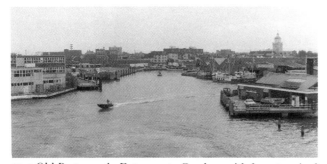

12.9 *Old Portsmouth. Entrance to Camber, with ferry terminal on left and Cathedral top right*

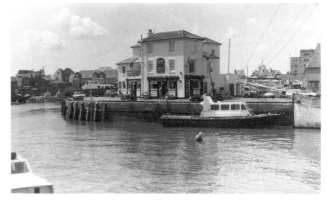

12.10 *Some yacht berths available in Camber after rounding the Bridge Tavern on the jetty*

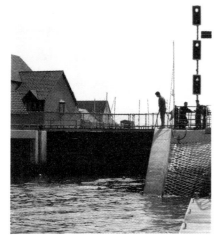

12.11 *Port Solent lock-gates with traffic signals and waiting pontoon*

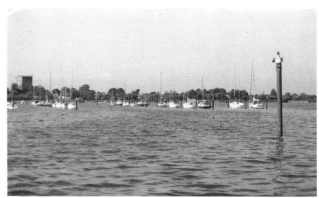

12.12 *Dredged channel leading outwards from Port Solent towards Portchester Castle. Note pile moorings on either side*

two is Fareham Lake. On the eastern side of the entrance to this creek there are three large big-ship mooring dolphins. A number of mooring buoys are placed on either side in the first reach, and above this the channel is marked by posts on the mud on either bank; R posts to port, G to starboard. Where the 2-mile long Portchester Channel joins the Fareham Channel, there is the R No. 57 porthand Bn (Fl R 10s.). At the end of the NNW channel – over 3 miles up – is the town of Fareham, but for a mile below this there is little water at low tide. This part of the channel between the R piles Nos. 18 and 19 is a prohibited anchorage, until the Reach bends to the NW for over $\frac{1}{2}$ mile before turning northward towards Fareham. The channel continues to be marked by piles. Yachts up to 1m8 draught can proceed to Fareham Quay 2 h. either side of HW after passing under power cables with 19m clearance below them.

Portchester Lake This is the eastern arm referred to above. It is a wide channel, running near the entrance in a NE direction, but there are several bends to be negotiated before it leads to the Port Solent marina, Portchester and the ruins of its castle. The navigation marks are the same as in Fareham Creek marked by R bns to port (seven with Fl G lts) and G bns to stb, nine with Fl R lts. The last half mile has only G lts.

Fountain Lake to the N and E of the Royal Dockyard is in constant use by continental ferries and should be used only by yachts with berths at the Whale Island naval sailing centre.

Signals Signals are displayed at Central Signal Station, Fort Blockhouse, or Gilkicker Signal Station or in HM ships as appropriate.

1. *Day.* R flag with W diagonal bar. *Night* R Lt over two G Lts Vert – no vessel is to leave the harbour or any of its creeks or lakes or approach N of Outer Spit buoy.

2. *Day.* R flag with W diagonal bar over one B ball – no vessel is to enter the harbour channel or approach channel from seaward. Outgoing vessels may proceed.

3. *Day.* One B ball over R flag with W diagonal bar – no vessel shall leave the harbour. Ingoing traffic may use the harbour channel and enter Portsmouth harbour.

4. *Day.* Large B pendant. *Night.* W Lt over two R Lts Vert – no vessel to anchor in the Man-of-War anchorages at Spithead.

5. *Day.* International Code Pendant superior to pendant zero – keep clear of HM ships under way.

6. *Day.* International Code Pendant superior to Pendant 9. *Night.* Three G Lts Vert. HM ship under way – give wide berth.

7. *Day.* International Code Pendant superior to Flags NE. *Night.* G over R Lt – proceed with great caution. Ships (other than car ferries) leaving Camber.

8. *Day.* Flag E. *Night.* R over amber Lt – submarine entering or leaving Haslar Lake. Keep clear.

9. *Day.* International Code Pendant superior to Flag A. *Night.* Two R Lts horizontal – have divers down.

10. IALA Port Movement signal Lts control traffic from Fort Blockhouse.

Anchorages, etc. Portsmouth Harbour and its approaches are under the jurisdiction of the Queen's Harbour Master, tel. 0705–82235, ext. 23694. Boats over 20m may not move without his permission on Ch 11 or 13.

(1) *Haslar Lake.* No room to anchor, bottom foul. Private moorings mostly for services personnel. Apply to RNSA, or Joint Services Sailing Centre adjacent Haslar Bridge, to ask whether a mooring may be temporarily vacant. Small power boats and shoal draught yachts with lowering masts can proceed under the bridge into Alverstoke Lake and anchor there.

(2) *Camper & Nicholson's Marina.* Enquire on VHF Ch 37 or at fuel pontoon, tel. 0705–524811. All facilities including building and repairs. Also moorings for very large yachts.

(3) Just above C. & N. Marina there are the Gosport Borough yacht moorings in *the Cold Harbour* with sets of double

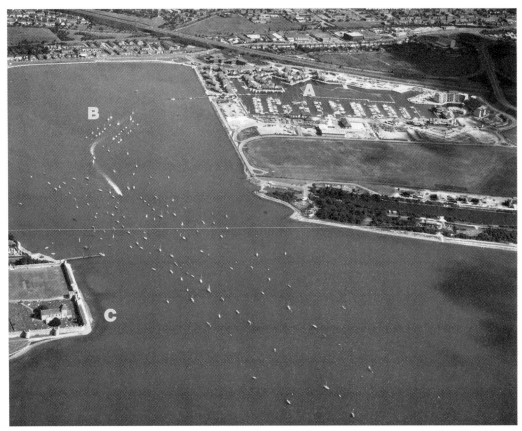

12.13 *Approach to Port Solent Marina (A) up the channel to the east of Portchester Castle (C), with final approach dredged to 1m5 (B)*

moorings let annually. Enquire at Gosport boatyard premises on the quay whether a set is temporarily vacant.

(4) *Gosport Cruising Club, Weevil Lake*. Apply at Club H.Q. boat for possible temporary mooring.

(5) *Hardway*. All available space occupied by moorings. Hardway Sailing club (tel. 581875) is hospitable and welcomes visitors from other clubs; it maintains a trot of five fore and aft visitors' moorings off the pontoon and can advise whether any other moorings are temporarily available. The public hard and pontoon landing stage are the only landing places in the vicinity. Club scrubbing piles and launching site, fuels, chandlery and inn are adjacent with short walk to boatyard, shops, restaurant and buses.

(6) On east side of harbour entrance is *The Camber*, a small commercial harbour with little room for visiting yachts. Permission to berth must first be obtained from the Dock Master at the entrance, Ch 11. Facilities within include yacht yards sailmaker and chandler.

(7) *Fareham Lake*. Anchorage now full of private moorings. Temporary moorings off Wicor Marine (and launching site near HW); enquire at yard (tel. 0329–237112) whether any mooring vacant. Near Fareham Quay, yacht builder, chandler, launching site at public slipway. Shops, banks, hotel, restaurants, etc. at Fareham. EC Wed. Station and buses.

(8) With reduction of danger area from Tipner Ranges, *Spider Lake and Bomb Ketch Lake* are now full of moorings but have no facilities – the nearest being at Hardway or Wicor.

(9) *Portchester*. Anchorage difficult as fairway must be kept clear and all available space near Portchester SC is occupied by moorings. Apply to duty officer at club for possibility of temporary mooring. If one is available, the historic castle will be found interesting and facilities are quite good. Club, inn, small shops, club scrubbing and launching site at Portchester hard but often fully booked up and hardly approachable at summer weekends. EC Tues, some Wed.

(10) *Portsmouth Cruising Club* has drying moorings and the usual facilities, but no shops near and $\frac{1}{2}$ mile (0.8 km) walk to buses.

(11) *Port Solent*. A major new marina complex for 850 boats including visitors. It is $3\frac{1}{4}$ miles from the entrance to Portsmouth Harbour along a well-marked channel dredged 1m5 below CD along last $\frac{1}{2}$ mile. Access 24h. Contact on Ch 37. Free flow through locks: at Springs $-2\frac{1}{2}$h. HW to $+3$h.; or $\pm$1h. at Neaps. Waiting area outside dredged 2mo. Waiting pontoons on either side of lock. Movements controlled by 3 Vert lights: GGW indicates two-way traffic with caution. Boats drawing up to 3m5 acceptable.

Facilities At Gosport and Portsmouth there are first-rate facilities and shops of every kind. EC Wed at both towns, Southsea Sat. Express rail service from Portsmouth Town or Harbour stations. Ferries and hovercraft to Ryde, I.W. Car ferries to Wootton, I.W., from Camber. Good bus services. Launching sites: (1) Portsmouth from car ferry slip provided ferries are not obstructed; the position is congested during the summer months. (2) From hard in Gosport Borough marina adjacent to Gosport boatyard office, with very limited public car parking near. (3) At hard of Gosport Cruising Club in Weevil Lake 3 hours either side of HW. New public dinghy landing on reclaimed section between C. & N. and Gosport Ferry pontoon. Yacht clubs: RNSA and R. Albert YC (0705–825924), Portsmouth SC (0705–820596), Hardway SC (0705–581875), Portsmouth Harbour CC (0705–664337), Portchester SC (0705–876375), Fareham S & MBC, (0329–80738). Port Solent has full facilities. Tel. (0705): Marina Control and enquiries 210765. Chandlery 219843. Restaurant 321025. Club/café 370164.

Weather See Chichester p. 90.

Southampton Weather Centre: 0703–228844.

13 Bembridge Harbour

Charts: BA 2022, 394 or 2050; Im 3; Stan 11

High Water   +00h. 14m. Dover.
Heights above Datum *in Harbour MHWS 3m1. MHWN 2m3. MLWS 0m3. MLWN 0m4.*
Depths   *There are extensive sands which dry at LW but a new 2m0 channel has been dredged (1990) to harbour entrance. Thence fairway to Brading Marina is 1m3 below CD. Water off new Bembridge Marina 1m8.*

BEMBRIDGE is a charming harbour at the east end of the Island. The marked channel is approached from the north and lies to the west of St Helen's Fort. The entrance itself is protected from westerly and southerly winds. The 2m0 dredged channel has transformed its appeal to visiting yachts.

Approach and Entrance   The approach to Bembridge Harbour is made from a NE direction to a yellow Bn (R ½ s.) with an X topmark 1 cable NW of St Helen's Fort (Fl 3 10s. 16m 8M). The Bn has a tide-gauge which indicates the least depth in the channel. It may be left on either hand before picking up the channel between the buoys, small G con to starboard and R cans to port on a SSW'ly course. Within the harbour gradually bear to starboard to pass between No. 13 G buoy and No. 10 R can buoy and then follow the buoyed channel to St Helen's.

Berths, Moorings and Anchorages   Anchoring within a cable of St Helen's Fort or inside the harbour is prohibited. Proceed up the buoyed fairway to St Helen's quay and marina, with 100 pontoon berths drawing 1m2 to 1m8 at Springs, or lie alongside the quay by arrangement and dry out where there is soft mud in parts. Do not secure at Bembridge SC pontoons but at the new marina immediately to the E where there are 60

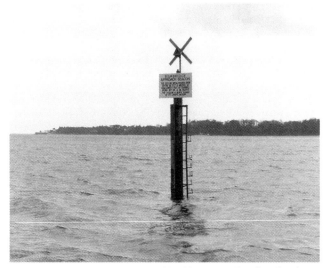

13.1 *Bembridge light beacon with tide gauge showing depth at shallowest part of channel*

visitors' berths alongside (1991).

Twin-keel shoal draught boats can dry out on the port hand of the entrance, on the beach near Bembridge Pt, but the beach is soon filled up at weekends during the season.

Otherwise moorings for visiting vessels are very limited and are all privately owned. Applications should be made before arrival on VHF Ch 37 or by telephone on 0983–874436 or through the HM on 0983–872828. Vessels should never pick up vacant moorings without prior arrangement.

Anchor north of St Helen's Fort to seaward of tide-gauge Bn

while waiting sufficient tide to enter the channel. In winds between W and S there is good anchorage eastward of Bembridge off Under Tyne outside local moorings, but the landing is rough and it is ½ mile walk to the harbour.

Facilities   There are several good yacht yards and marine engineers. Water by hose and fuel at marina, with Brading Harbour YC adjacent (which welcomes temporary members); shops and PO ¼ mile distant at St Helen's. Diesel oil is also supplied by Harbour Engineering at the sheds ¼ mile east of BHYC and both diesel and petrol at their embankment premises next to Coombes yard. There are hotels and restaurants, small shops. EC Thurs. Buses to all parts of the Island. Sandown airfield close. Launching sites at concrete ramp near St Helen's seamark, or by arrangement with yards or clubs. Yacht clubs: Bembridge SC, Brading Harbour YC.

Weather   See Chichester, see p. 90.
Southampton Weather Centre, tel. 0703–228844.

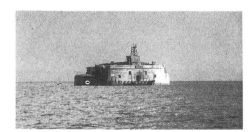

13.2 *St Helen's Fort*

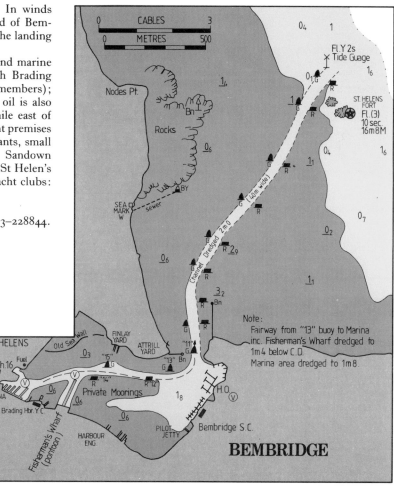

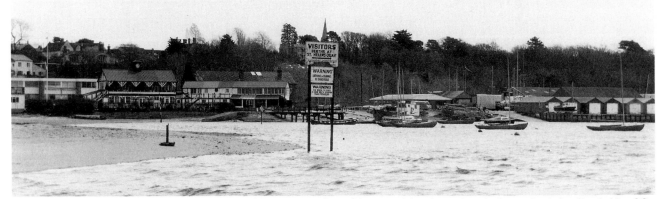

13.3 *Bembridge Point. Plans for 1990 include building new marina with some visitors' moorings in front of existing Bembridge SC, whose clubhouse will be re-located in place of hutted stores on right*

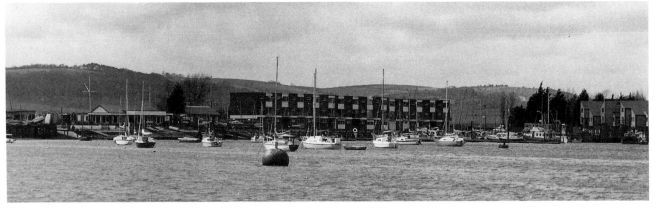

13.4 *Fairway in Brading Harbour towards St Helen's Quay and Marina (far right)*

14 Wootton Creek

Charts: BA 2022; Im Y20; Stan 11

High Water *+00h. 14m. Dover.*
Heights above Datum *MHWS 4m5. MLWS 0m7. MHWN 3m6. MLWN 1m7.*
Depths *The channel is dredged to 3m0 up to the ferry slipway. Basin dries LAT on soft mud. In the river there is only 0m6 to 0m3.*

WOOTTON CREEK is a pretty but overcrowded harbour shared by yachts and the Fishbourne car ferries. The entrance is normally easy to identify and navigate.

Approach and Entrance The entrance to the Creek is clearly marked by the Wootton Bn, half a mile offshore, a BY N-cardinal pile (Q W). The narrow channel dredged to 3m0 has its own Oc WRG 10s. sector light at the inshore end of the ferry terminal. The W sector is on 225° down the middle of the fairway, marked on its starboard hand by three lit G dolphins (G (2) G 5s., G 3s. and Q G in succession). It is very busy in summer months. Ferries have absolute right of way. When the yacht comes to the third dolphin she may stand on for the end of the ferry pier, leaving this very close to port and with sufficient rise of tide enter the bight situated to the NW of the ferry pier. Here she will find moorings belonging to the Royal Victoria YC with Berthing Master in attendance. Visiting yachtsmen are welcome. To sail up the river proceed from No. 3 dolphin, turning slowly to starboard on the 270° transit of leading marks, which consist of two W triangles on the W foreshore near a boathouse. The channel is marked by G buoys to starboard and R buoys to port round the next bend. The channel is narrow, and strangers should be careful not to run on to or cross the finger of mud shown on the harbour plan on the port side of the channel between the Creek channel and the bight moorings. A

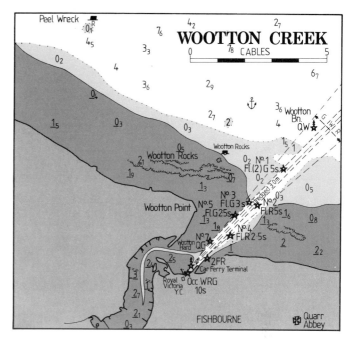

R buoy sits on this spit. There are a slip and a dinghy park on the starboard side of the Creek just S of the boatyards.

Lights The N-cardinal Wootton Bn has a Q No. 1 Bn is Fl (2) G 5s.; No. 2 is Fl R 5s.; No. 3 is W Fl G 3s.; No. 4 is Q R; No. 5 is Q G.

Anchorage There is reasonable anchorage in settled weather and offshore winds outside the Creek to NW of Wootton Bn at the entrance. Within the Creek the only anchorage for boats drawing up to 1m5 lies in the bight beyond the ferry pier, well clear of the ferries' approach and turning area. Here it dries out at LAT, but yachts sit upright in very soft mud. Anchors should be buoyed. There are also many moorings but it is best to obtain advice from the Berthing Master, who usually meets incoming yachts and directs them to a berth. He can be contacted by phone on 0983–882325.

Shallow draught vessels, which can take the mud, will find room to anchor up-river as far as the pub at Wootton Bridge, but there are many moorings in the best parts.

Facilities At Fishbourne there are an inn and garage, and the R. Victoria YC clubhouse. This club has good facilities with hard, car park, changing rooms, bar and club boatman. Visiting yachts are welcome and temporary membership is available to members of recognized yacht clubs. (Tel. 0983–882325). At Wootton, $\frac{3}{4}$ mile up the river or a mile's walk from Fishbourne, there are three boatyards, garage (water and petrol), PO, shops, inn. EC Thurs. Launching sites: from ferry hard or YC by arrangement. Frequent buses from Wootton Bridge to Ryde and Newport.

Weather See Chichester p. 90.

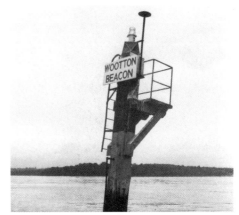

14.1 *Wootton Beacon at seaward end of the approach channel to Fishbourne*

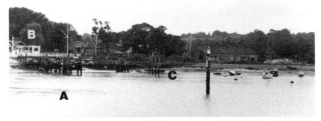

14.2 *(A) Approach towards old ferry ramp (B) R Victoria YC (C) Yacht Club pontoon*

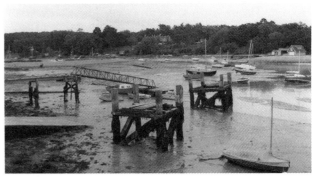

14.3 *Low water at Yacht Club pontoon, showing channel towards upper reaches of Wootton Creek*

15 Cowes

Charts: BA 2793; IM Y20; Stan 11

High Water +ooh. 14m. Dover.
Heights above Datum MHWS 4m2. MLWS om6. MHWN 3m5. MLWN 1m7.
Depths The River Medina has a least depth of 3m0 in the fairway from the entrance to E Cowes ferry terminal, then 2m1 as far as Medham, ½ mile short of the Folly Inn, when depths reduce to om6, getting steadily shallower thereafter. At Springs the river dries out on the last 1¼ miles to Newport.

COWES is famous as the leading yacht racing centre in the world, and is the headquarters of the Royal Yacht Squadron. It is a town of tradition and character that time has little changed and is the most conveniently placed harbour in the Solent. The harbour is well protected except from the N and NE in which case it is wise to seek shelter up-river.

Approach and Entrance The entrance is narrow but well marked. The fairway lies on the W side of the entrance, and is marked by the porthand R (No. 4) light buoy (Q R 5m) and the unlit starboard-hand G Con (No. 3) buoy; in the harbour there are two R porthand buoys of which No. 8 is Fl (2) R 5s.

Approaching from the E, to clear the Shrape Mud near LW steer to Trinity House buoy (Fl Y 2s.) and then keep on the line from the buoy to the N of the conspicuous Royal Yacht Squadron castle until the fairway is entered. A long breakwater extends across the Shrape bank, affording some shelter from the NE. The projected new Port Medina marina with its considerable reclamation and dredging programme will probably have a consequential effect on the depths over the Shrape. There is little water to the N of this breakwater, and the temptation to cut across towards W Cowes must be resisted unless the tide permits.

Coming from the W, there is deep water a cable offshore but there are ledges of rock E of Egypt Point and off the shore along Cowes Green to the Royal Yacht Squadron. Leave No. 3 outer G buoy to starboard. Note that an early ebb which runs contrary to the main tide will be found between Egypt Point and the Royal Yacht Squadron 1h. before HW Dover. Tides run up to 3½ kts across the entrance.

There is a speed limit of 6 kts.

Lights The BY north cardinal Prince Consort buoy, NE of the entrance, exhibits a Q W Lt, and there is a Lt (Q R 5M) on the outer (No. 4) porthand buoy. A QR Lt is at the end of the eastern breakwater. Leading lights on 164° are: Front Iso 2s., Rear Iso R 2s. The rear R Lt is visible 120° to 240°. The principal lights in

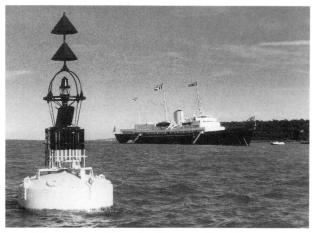

15.1 *Prince Consort N-cardinal buoy, half a mile north of entrance to Medina River*

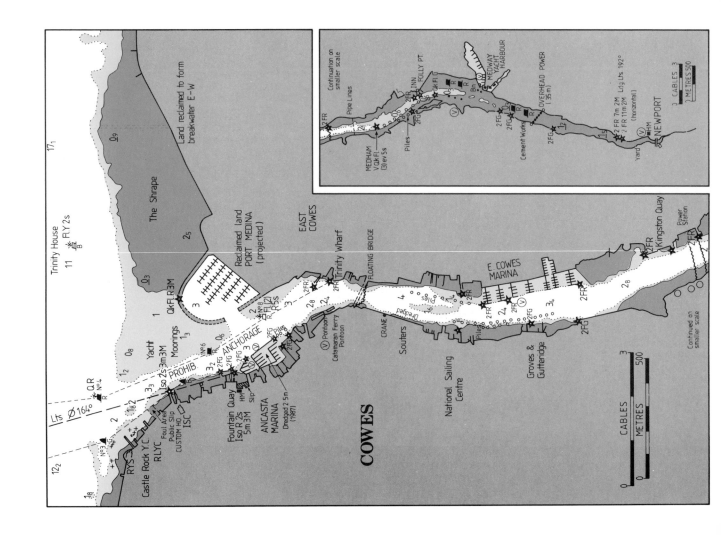

the River Medina are shown on the harbour plan.

Anchorage, Moorings and Marinas Large yachts anchor or moor on buoys provided in the roads north of the Shrape bank or outboard of the Ancasta Marina pontoons. Smaller yachts anchor on the Shrape well to the NW of the breakwater and local moorings in positions depending upon their draught, remembering that at MLWS there is om6 and at MLWN 1m7 more water than shown at chart datum. Anchor should be buoyed to avoid fouling mooring chains.

Four large visitors' moorings are laid off Cowes esplanade for temporary use. There are many private moorings in The Hole on the E side of the harbour and NW of it. Additional moorings are laid for the various classes of competitors in Cowes Week and the many other regattas regularly held there. None should be picked up without permission of the HM, on Ch 16, 6, 11 or by telephone at 0983–293952.

In strong northerly winds, it is better to enter one of the marinas or proceed up the river beyond the floating bridge where there are pile moorings for visiting yachts of any size. The floating bridge guards Ch 10.

The Ancasta Marina on the old Groves & Gutteridge site just upstream of the Red Funnel pontoon ferry has 130 berths and a planned minimum depth of 2m4. During major international events like the Admiral's Cup most of the berths in the sheltered northern end of the marina are not available for visitors, while the majority of the rest are held by long-term berth-holders. So visitors may find themselves outboard of the outer N-S pontoon run, lying as many as eight abreast, with all the attendant worries of clashing rigs and cruising boats wanting to extricate themselves from the trots to catch the tide during the small hours. Immediately upstream there are piles and mooring buoys available and a new long pontoon with 2m0 outboard with its

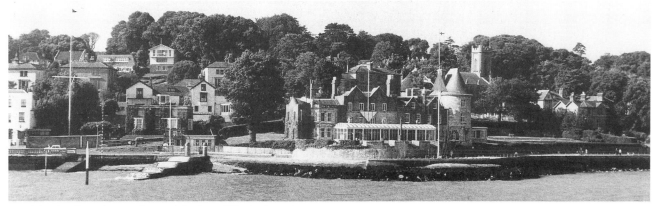

15.2 *The Castle at Cowes, home of the Royal Yacht Squadron. White twin-gabled building and flagstaff above landing-steps is the Castle Rock Yacht Club*

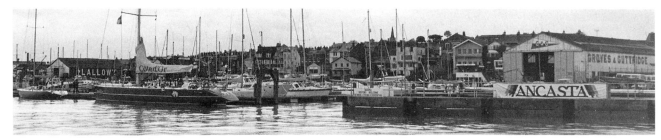

15.3 *Entrance to Ancasta Marina upstream from Red Funnel ferry pier*

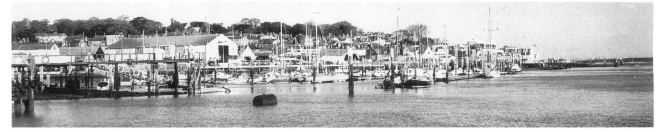

15.4 *Ancasta Marina facing downstream*

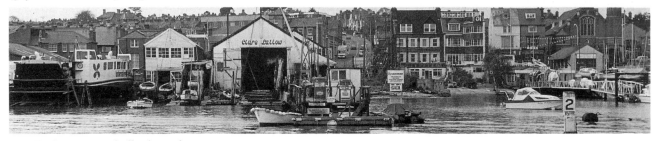

15.5 *Fuel pontoon at Lallow's yard*

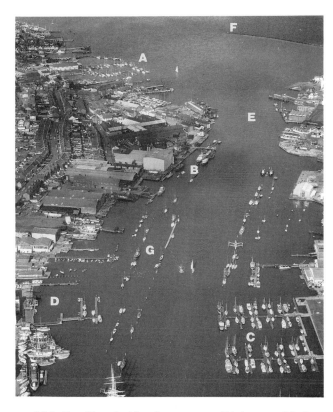

15.6 *Medina River looking downstream. (A) Ancasta Marina (B) Souter's Yard (C) East Cowes Marina (D) National Sailing School (E) Chain Ferry (F) East Cowes breakwater (G) Fore-and-aft pile moorings*

own walkway ashore opposite the old hovercraft apron, which is now a thriving DIY boatyard with tools for rental. Visiting yachts may touch down there free of charge, but not lie overnight without the HM's permission. The inshore side of this pontoon is reserved for dinghies and tenders, tel. 0983–295724. VHF Ch 37.

Port Medina. A new 550-berth marina with least depth of 2m5 is planned for E Cowes, based on the site of the Westland Hovercraft factory and by reclaiming and dredging part of the Shrape. The breakwater will be extended anticlockwise from NW to SW, giving some much needed added protection to the Ancasta Marina in W Cowes.

The East Cowes Marina is located 3 cables beyond the floating bridge on the port hand. It has 220 alongside berths in depths of 2–3m at its outer end. If you can come to terms with being on the wrong side of the floating bridge and dependent on launches to take you to West Cowes where the action is, it has the advantage of generally available berths and complete shelter from winds from any quarter. Tel. 0983–293983.

The depths in the Medina above the floating bridge are as shown on the harbour plan or, in greater detail, on Admiralty chart 2793 or Imray Y20. At low water there is at least 2m1 as far as Medham Bn 4 cables beyond Kingston Quay on the E bank. There are continuous pile moorings on each side of the fairway. Those available for visitors are clearly indicated.

Off the Folly Inn there are 12 pile moorings in 0m6 which has 1m4 at MLWS or 2m3 at MLWN. The Inn has its own landing pontoon, with 1m0 at MLWS, a restaurant and village shop. It is the home of the locals' most popular event afloat – the Folly Regatta.

The Medina Marina has been excavated from land on the same side of the river. It has a clearly marked R and G channel and a conspicuous harbour control tower which listens out on Ch 37. Once inside there are 220 berths for yachts drawing up to

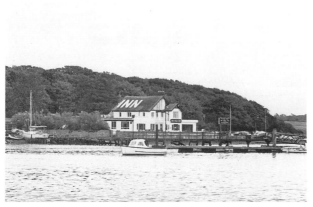

15.7 *Folly Inn and pontoon half-way to Newport*

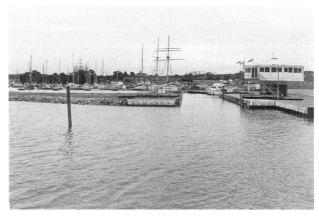

15.8 *Entrance to Medina Yacht Harbour, lock-gates open*

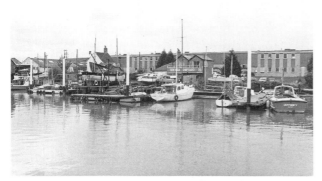

15.9 *Odessa Shipyard in Newport on the west bank*

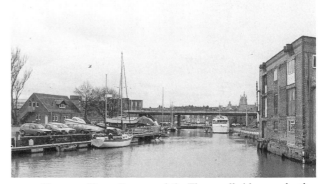

15.10 *Newport Town Quay on left. The roadbridge marks the limit of navigable water*

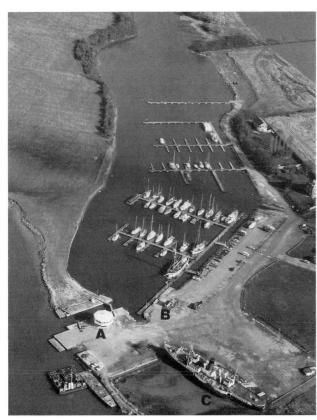

15.11 *Medina Marina half a mile upstream from the Folly Inn. (A) Harbour Office (B) Fuel berth (C) 'Medway Queen' restaurant*

2mo, fuel, water, shore power and a good restaurant on the old paddlewheel steamer *Medway Queen* berthed next door. Tel. 0983–526733.

Newport provides alongside berths for boats which can dry out right in the heart of the picturesque old town. The tidal restriction is not quite so daunting as the charts indicate. The depth of water alongside at Newport is always 4ft. less than that showing on the tide-gauge at the upstream end of the Red Funnel ferry pontoon. The pattern of the tide encourages a visit long enough for lunch ashore even if you draw 1m8 and don't want to take the mud. The ebb starts 20 minutes before HW Cowes, runs for half an hour, then stands for 2 h. only 1ft. below HW level. The upper reaches of the river are well marked by channel buoys. If in doubt, contact the HM Newport on 0983–525994.

Facilities It is hard to conceive of any requirement for yachtsmen which is not catered for. In particular the new-look Ancasta Marina has put on a permanent basis many of the facilities formerly provided in tents or caravans during regattas. There are yacht yards of international repute, with slips and hoists capable of handling boats close to maxi size, sailmakers, electronics engineers, the best rigger in the world, brokers, yacht chandlers, hotels and restaurants, Customs, bonded stores and many shops of all kinds including yachting outfitters. EC Wed. Bus connections to all parts. Ferry and hydrofoil services to Southampton. Yacht clubs: Royal Yacht Squadron, R. London YC, R. Corinthian YC, Island SC, East Cowes SC, Cowes Corinthian YC. Launching sites: (1) From the slipway off the esplanade near Island SC, with car park adjacent. (2) From the slipway on town quay adjacent to the ferry pontoon, but car parking restricted. (3) Heavy boats can be craned into the water from Thetis jetty or at Souter's by arrangement.

Weather See Chichester p. 90.

Southampton Weather Centre 0703–228844.

16　Hamble River

Charts: BA 2022; Im C3; Stan 11

Double High Water *First HW Springs approx. −00h. 20m. Dover.*
Heights above Datum *at Calshot Castle MHWS 4m4. MLWS 0m6. MHWN 3m6. MLWN 1m8.*
Depths *3m6 in entrance, and upwards of 2m1 in the channel as far as Mercury Yacht Harbour. Above this 1m5 will be found to Bursledon bridge, and in parts this depth is exceeded.*

APART FROM the Elephant Yard at Bursledon and the riverside Jolly Sailor pub next door, allowing the soap opera 'Howard's Way' the slender pretext of having something to do with yachting, the HAMBLE RIVER's popularity rests on its providing over 3,000 secure berths for keelboats; half of them are alongside well-appointed efficiently run marinas, all readily accessible from seaward at any state of wind or tide. It is also only 1½ h. by road from London to this excellent jumping-off point for cruising or racing anywhere. Maintenance, supply and repair facilities match the social amenities in hospitable yacht clubs, real pubs and restaurants at either end of the gastronomic range. Although visitors' berths are always available on the piles or at the marinas, don't count on picking up a long-term arrangement, for there are few vacancies. The river is packed as far as Bursledon bridge and beyond.

Approach and Entrance　Coming from seaward, get Calshot Castle abeam and then alter to 350° to leave the G Hook pillar buoy (Q G bell) to starboard and head for the S-cardinal Hamble Point buoy (Q (6) LF 15s.) to pass it close to port on course 345°. From here on there's shoal water close at hand on either side – some of the channel marking piles dry out at

MLWS. By day the transit is No. 6 R pile and a conspicuous red roof in the trees ashore. The red roof is not easy to pick out, particularly in summer. A better transit is to take the left-hand edge of the boat park at Point Hamble in line with No. 4 pile. By night No. 6 is Oc (2) R 12s. in line with the West Hamble beacon (Q R 12m). From here on the channel is marked by R and G piles, most of them lit, as shown on the plan.

Between the unlit No. 4 R pile and No. 5 G, alter to starboard to pick up the 026° transit for final approach. By day it is not easy to pick up the BW chequered Bn in front and the one on Warsash SC beyond, so just sail to keep the G No. 7 and 9 piles to starboard and pass outside the end of the long Navigation School pier. At night these lights are easy enough to pick up (Q G in transit with Iso G 6s.).

At the Warsash Shore Bn swing to port on a NNW heading and proceed up-river between piles and moorings as shown on the harbour plans. Speed limit 6 knots, enforced.

Anchorage and Berths　To all intents and purposes there is no room left in the river for anchoring, except by shoal draught boats off the fairway. Application can be made to the HM at Warsash on Ch 16 or 68 or by telephone to (Locks Heath) 04895–6387. Visitors can also land at his pontoon in front of the Rising Sun pub for advice. In the summer he is usually afloat in his launch. He may direct visitors as follows:

1. *Warsash.* Piles in mid-stream off the Hamble Point Marina.
2. *Off Port Hamble.* Pile moorings on the E side of the fairway. In each case some piles are clearly designated for other users than visiting yachts.
3. *Hamble Point, Port Hamble, Mercury and Swanwick Marinas* usually have vacant berths for short-stay visitors. They can be called on VHF Ch 37. Their touch-down berths for visitors seeking further instructions are clearly indicated.

Facilities　Customs office at Port Hamble Marina, tel. 0703–452007 where bonded stores can be arranged. Water, fuel,

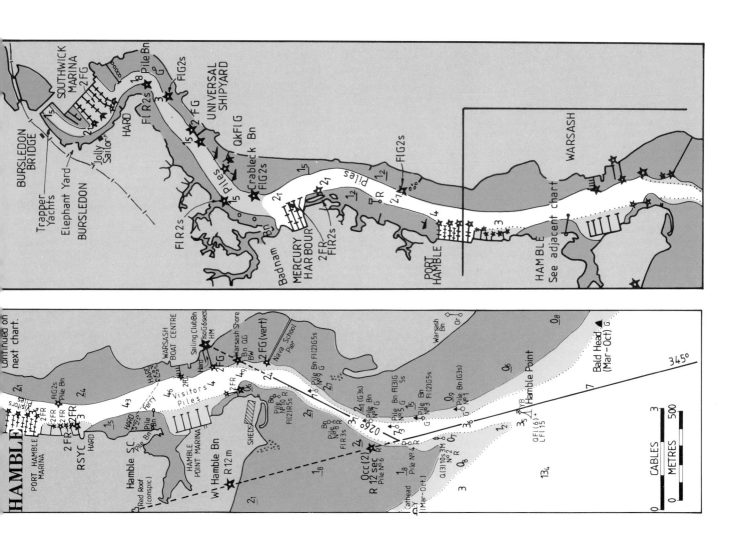

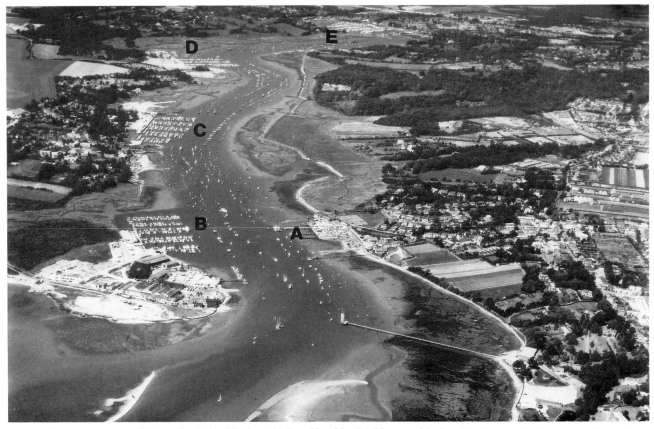

16.1 *(A) Harbour Master (B) Hamble Point Marina (C) Port Hamble (D) Mercury Marina (E) Swanwick Marina at Moody's yard (Aerofilms Ltd)*

garbage disposal and shore power at all marinas and yards. Builders of 12-metre, high-performance luxury powerboats and a wide range of stock auxiliary sailing boats at Warsash, Hamble, Swanwick and Bursledon. Each has its own chandlery, marine and electronic engineers for supply or repair. Travel-hoist at Swanwick big enough for a maxi. Slipways at all yards and marinas. Three hards available for DIY scrubbing against piles: Warsash, Mercury, and the hard opposite Swanwick Marina and the old Mercury jetty. Sailmakers at Sarisbury (Bruce Banks Ltd) and J. R. Williams at Hamble. Proctors Metal Masts at Swanwick. Banks at Hamble and Warsash. Restaurants, shops and POs at Hamble, Warsash, Bursledon and Swanwick. EC Wed. Except Warsash Thurs. Hotel and restaurant Hamble, Warsash and Bursledon. Launching sites:

(1) Warsash public hard, car park adjacent.

(2) Hamble public hard, car park adjacent.

(3) Swanwick Shore public hard (next to Moody's yacht yard) with car park adjacent.

(4) At Bursledon on SW side of bridge and at Land's End public hard with car park at the station ¼ mile distant. Buses from Warsash, Hamble, Swanwick and Bursledon. Station at Bursledon. Southampton Airport at Eastleigh. Yacht clubs: R. Southern YC, Hamble River SC, RAF YC, Warsash SC.

Weather   See Chichester p. 90.
Southampton Weather Centre tel. 0703–228844.
BBC Radio Solent 300m 221m 0745.

17   Southampton

Charts: BA 1905, 2041; Im C3

Double High Water   *First HW Springs −00h. 13m. Dover. 'Young Flood' stand lasts from 1½ to 3h. after local LW.*
Heights above Datum   *MHWS 4m7 MLWS 0m5. MHWN 3m7. MLWN 1m9.*
Depths   *Deep channels dredged 10m to W Docks, thereafter shelving in the Rivers Test and Itchen.*

SOUTHAMPTON WATER is a 6-mile long straight fairway from Calshot Castle to the Royal Pier from where the Red Funnel ferries sail. It is dredged to 10m along a well-buoyed and lit fairway. The days when it was the greatest passenger liner port in the world are gone for ever. So has all the cross-Channel ferry traffic and a significant slice of the container trade. Nowadays the largest ships regularly visiting Southampton are tankers which stop at the oil jetties at Fawley. Until recently it has had little to offer visiting yachtsmen, other than being a convenient point to pick up or drop crews, although there are some moorings on either side of the fairway, mostly for local owners. The picture has changed dramatically, with three new marinas within ready access of the fast rail and motorway networks which serve Southampton so well. It is on the way to becoming a home for big yachts once again.

All traffic in Southampton Water is monitored and controlled. Local bye-laws requiring small craft and yachts of all sizes to give way to steamships are strictly enforced.

Approach and Entrance   When entering Southampton Water the main channel lies between Calshot Spit Lt float (Fl 5s.) and the N-cardinal BY pillar buoy (Q) thence running NW close to Calshot Castle and its conspicuous radar tower.

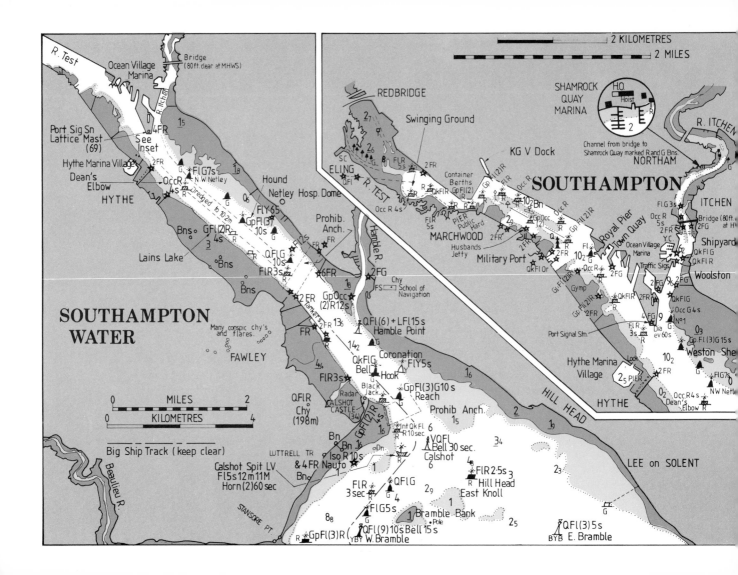

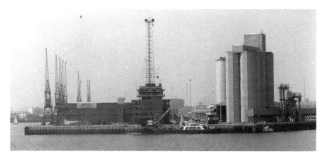

17.1 *Port Signal and Radar station at the division of Southampton Water with River Test to the left, Itchen River to the right*

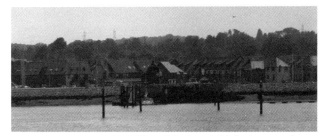

17.2 *Approach to Hythe Village Marina, with lock-gates shut*

Approaching from the eastward, keep well offshore between Hill Head and Hamble, as the shoal water extends a surprisingly long way from the shore. Whether coming from E or W remember the Bramble Bank, situated in mid-Solent. In spite of being such a well-known danger, yachts still go aground on this shingle shoal which may vary from year to year in depth and position. At the lowest Springs it used to be the scene of an annual cricket match organized by Uffa Fox.

Once within Southampton Water navigation is easy. Mud flats run off a long way on both sides. The deep ship channel is dredged to 10m2 and marked by Fl R can buoys on the west side, and by Fl G conical buoys on the east side.

The docks will be seen from afar, with the conspicuous Port Signal and Radar Station at the junction of two channels, the Test river leading approximately NW, and the Itchen river joining from NNE. The Test is the clearly-marked channel leading past the Ocean Dock, the Royal Pier and the long line of the Western Docks to the container berths.

If proceeding to moorings farther up the **River Test**, the Marchwood Channel may be taken. The entrance lies just N of the Middle Swinging Ground No. 2 R can buoy about 3 cables WNW of the Royal pier. The leading Bns will then be brought into transit at 298°. The front one is a W triangle on a dolphin and the rear a W diamond on a dolphin. The depth on the transit is 2m4 to within ½ cable of the front Bn. Close to starboard lies a long shoal marked on its far NE side by a Bn and a pile. On the port hand from No. 2 buoy to Marchwood buoy there is shoal water almost as far as Husband's jetty, where it deepens to 2m and more for 3 cables. Observing a N-cardinal buoy (Q W) close SW of No. 2 buoy will keep you in the channel. There are a great many moorings in this area. The shoal area in the Marchwood Channel lies from about ½ cable SE of the first Bn nearly as far as the rear Bn and both Bns should be left close to port. There are many small craft moorings in the area in depths of 0m5 to 0m9. Immediately after passing the rear Bn a vessel is in deep water of the main channel dredged to 10m2, leading past the container berths and Swinging Ground.

The Eling Channel, which is very narrow and dries out, is entered close S to the NW Swinging Ground (Eling) buoy. It is marked by Bns with triangle topmarks on the starboard hand

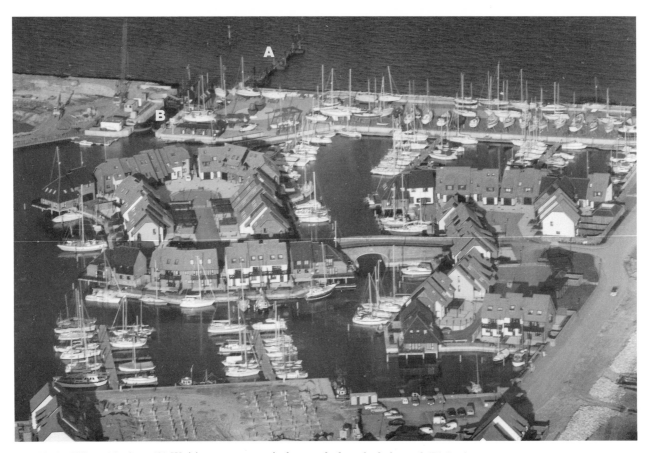

17.3 *Hythe Village Marina. (A) Waiting pontooon at inshore end of marked channel (B) Lock*

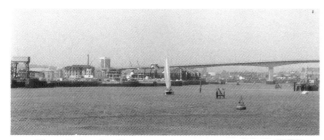

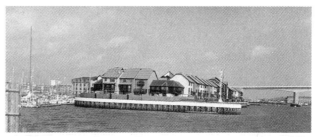

17.4 *River Itchen leading towards entrance to Ocean Village Marina, just right of yacht under sail*

17.5 *Entrance to Ocean Village Marina from Itchen River Traffic signals on beacon at north side of entrance (RRR: all stop; GGW: free flow either direction)*

except at the junction with the Redbridge Channel, which is marked by a YB S-cardinal junction Bn. Near the entrance of Eling Channel there are two porthand Bns, S of which there are small craft moorings in 0m3. Power cables cross the channel, height 36m.

The River Itchen and Approaches The last starboard-hand buoy before entering the river is Weston Shelf (Fl (3) G 15s.) to seaward of the drying flats which it marks. On the W shore is Hythe Pier from which small harbour ferries run across to Southampton. Immediately upstream of the pierhead is an E-cardinal BYB buoy (Q (3) W 10s.) marking the entrance to Hythe Village Marina.

The deep channel up the river goes close by the docks on its W shore. The last entrance on the port hand before reaching the 80-ft centre span of the Woolston bridge is into Ocean Village Marina, developed on the site left after the big RO/RO ferries mostly moved to Portsmouth.

Passing under the bridge, the channel still favours the western bank, with depths down to 2m6. Strong tides may be encoun-

tered in this stretch of the river, running up to $3\frac{1}{2}$ knots on the ebb at Springs. Half a mile upstream Camper & Nicholson's old yard is now the Shamrock Quay Marina, where every conceivable amenity awaits yachtsmen of all tastes.

Port Signal and Radar Station Call sign 'SPR' (Southampton Port Radio) is available for communication on VHF Channels 16, 14 and 12. Harbour Office tel. 0703–330022.

Anchorages Where available these are generally remote from commercial activities, but it is possible in suitable weather conditions to anchor anywhere that can be found in Southampton Water clear of (a) prohibited areas, (b) shipping fairways and docks and their approaches and (c) moorings. The anchor should be buoyed. A riding light is necessary at night. Some of the positions for anchorage or moorings are:

(1) *Between Calshot Castle and Fawley R buoy* temporary anchorage off the mud flat in moderate W to SW winds.

(2) *Hythe.* Large yachts lie S of Hythe pier. For smaller craft enquire at yacht yard or club for moorings, or anchor south of the pier. Yacht yard, hotel, shops, petrol, etc. EC. Wed.

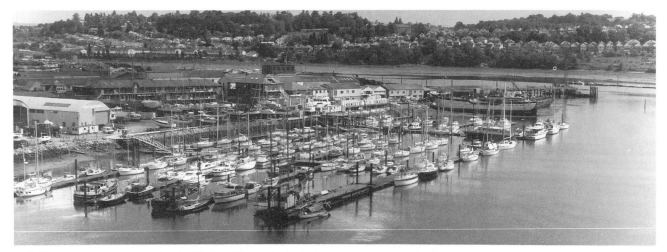

17.6 *Shamrock Quay on west bank of Itchen River, above the bridge*

(3) *Southampton.* There are Harbour Board moorings for large yachts off the Royal pier.

(4) *Marchwood.* Many moorings S of the Marchwood Channel. Enquire at Husband's shipyard or Marchwood YC. Fuel and water at shipyard jetty; frequent launches to Southampton Town Quay.

(5) *Container Swinging Ground.* Anchorage prohibited but at Neaps there is just room to anchor close beyond No. 14 and the Eling buoys.

(6) *River Itchen.* There are a few Harbour Board moorings for large yachts. Anchorage is possible in the Itchen River on the starboard hand out of the main fairway.

(7) *Netley.* Between the hard ½ mile NW of Netley dome and the

G and Y Bns marking a sewage outfall, but it is on a lee shore in the prevailing winds.

Alongside berths in marinas

Hythe Village. The entrance is just upstream of Hythe ferry pier. The seaward end of the short approach channel is marked by the E-cardinal buoy mentioned above, paired with a R can (Fl R (2) 5s.). The least depth outside the lock-gates is 2m. The gates are marked to seaward by 2F R and 2F G (vert). They are normally open for two-way traffic two hours either side of HW. There is a waiting pontoon on the port hand just outside. Call the HM on Ch 37, and he will direct visitors to an available berth. Traffic is governed by light signals (R for Stop; G for Go and 2R over G for free-flow traffic either way). Once inside the marina, there is a least depth of 2m5. Fuel, shore power and all normal marina facilities are on tap. The village of Hythe is only 10 minutes' walk away. Tel. 0703–849263. 180 berths + 50 for visitors.

Ocean Village. Opposite Vospers old yard there is a 450-berth yacht harbour (+50 for visitors) with a least depth of 2m0 and some berths considerably deeper – a J-Class berth is available there. It has the beauty of being easily accessible day or night at any state of the tide. Among many other amenities now located there, it is the home of the R. Southampton YC. Call on Ch 37 during daylight hours or by telephone to 0703–229461 or 228353. The Harbour Board's floating 200-ton crane can be deployed there, in case you want to lift a maxi or even bigger yacht. Charter yachts available. IALA traffic lights on N side of entrance 3FR = all stop, GGW = free flow.

Shamrock Quay. At Northam above Woolston bridge has only 220 berths, but keeps 40 free for visitors. Ashore it is a nautical Disneyland, on top of providing all technical and professional support needed for any boat. There is ample hard-standing for winter storage and refits, tel. 0703–229461.

As with the new-look Brighton Marina, property development is the primary aim of all three of Southampton's exciting new marinas. So if you want a waterside home or office overlooking your boat in that area, just say the word – and reach for your cheque-book.

Facilities Southampton provides facilities of every kind for yachts, large or small. Ministry of Transport office. Customs and bonded stores. Marine engineers, yacht agents, chart agency, compass adjusting, instruments and chandlery and smaller yards and boat-builders. Shops of all kinds. EC Mon. Some Wed. Hotels, restaurants, car ferry service, hydrofoil to Cowes. Good train services including express 70 minutes to London. Buses to all parts.

Launching sites
(1) From foreshore N of Hythe pier,
(2) from ramp at head of Ashlett Creek, S of oil refineries,
(3) from hard on N shore of Eling Creek,
(4) Itchen River at Woolston hard on E side or at both marinas,
(5) at public hard, Netley.
Yacht clubs: R. Southampton YC, Southampton SC, Eling SC, Weston SC, Hythe SC, Marchwood YC, Esso SC, Netley Cliff SC.

Weather   Local shipping forecasts from Southampton
Weather Centre 0703–228844.
Marinecall 0898–500467 or 500403.
Radio Solent (999 or 1359 kHz) at 0745 Mon-Fri,
0835 and frequently at weekends.
Niton VHF Ch 28 at 0833 and 2033.

*18 Beaulieu River

Charts: BA 2021; Im Y20; Stan 11

Double High Water at entrance. *First HW Springs −00h. 30m. Dover.*
Heights above Datum at entrance approx. *MHWS 3m7. MLWS 0m6. MHWN 3m1. MLWN 1m6.*

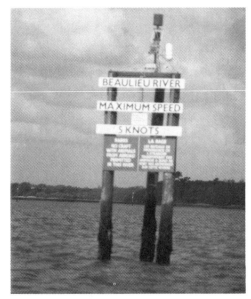

18.1 *Beacon marking entrance to Beaulieu River*

Depths *About 0m6 on the bar at LAT. Boats drawing 2m0 in strong seas or within 1 h. of MLWS should not attempt to enter. Since the Swash has been sealed off at Need's Oar, HW has been held up for an extra 45 mins, and the ebb runs for only 3¾ h. Within the river, depths are as on plan. There is a least depth of 1m8 up to the marina at Buckler's Hard, except at extreme LAT. At HW the river is navigable all the way to Beaulieu.*

BEAULIEU RIVER is the most beautiful anchorage within the Solent. A long, straight channel leads between the mud flats to the river proper, most of which lies between deep woods on either hand. Four miles upstream lies the historic village of Beaulieu, with its thirteenth-century Abbey and twentieth century motor museum. The entrance is shallow but marked, and available to most vessels except at exceptionally low spring tides.

Approach and Entrance From the W follow the line of the Hampshire coast, keeping ½ mile off the mud flats, until the R tripod Bn (R 5s. 3m) at the eastern end of Beaulieu Spit, the Lepe Coastguard cottages and a conspicuous white boathouse have been identified. Continue until the leading marks come into line at 339°. The shallowest part of the approach channel is to seaward of the dolphin, so at LW pick up the transit line of two O boards and keep it open to port, as the bar has recently shifted. The front is a board with triangular top on the first porthand pile (No. 2), and the rear, which is situated among dark-green trees, has a similar board with a triangular top but with a Vert B stripe in its centre. Do not confuse it with the RW diamond-topped telephone Bn 2 cables farther W. Keep close to the E of the transit and leave the dolphin to port across bar with 0m6. Within the entrance the river soon deepens and it is marked by R piles with can tops and R reflectors (even numbers) on the port hand and G piles (odd numbers) with conical tops and G reflectors to starboard (Nos. 5, 9 and 19 G Bns have lts G

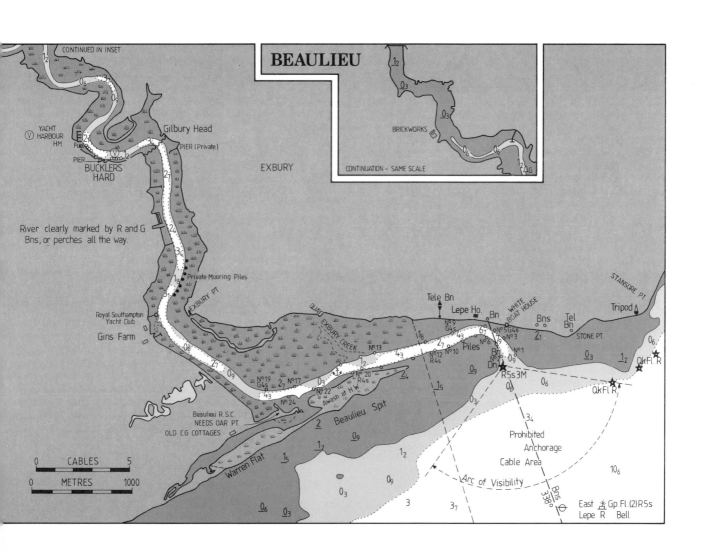

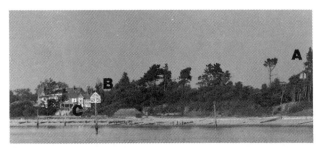

18.2 *With shoal water often shifting, in 1990 the best water was found on a transit of right-hand edge of Lepe House (C) with the front orange board on pile (B) on course 330°, as against recommended 338° transit of (A) and (B)*

4s.; Nos. 12 and 20 R Bns are R 4s.). Between Bns 4 and 6 there is a sharp bend to the WSW. Since the Swatchway or Bull Run was filled and closed in 1986 the ebb runs stronger in the river and sweeps across the channel to the SE between Bns 10 and 12.

From the eastward leave the three Q R Bns off Stone Point to starboard and do not steer direct to Beaulieu Spit dolphin near LW Springs, but steer to come on the leading transit 2 cables S of the Bn.

Once beyond the first bend the channel continues to be marked by pile Bns and it is fairly wide to the next bend at Need's Oar Point. From here the river is marked by perches, some of them inconspicuous and unpainted. There are a few shoal patches, as shown on the chart, which require attention at LW springs but, at most states of the tide, vessels of 2m0 draft have no difficulty in sailing up to the Yacht Harbour at Buckler's Hard and one mile beyond it.

The channel sweeps wide towards the E bank at the first bend after the marina, but at the next curve to port there is a spit out

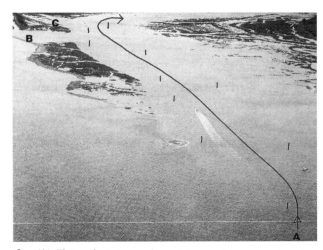

18.3 *(A) Channel upstream from entrance between red and green beacons (B) Former Swatchway blocked off (C) Need's Oar Point, site of Beaulieu River Sailing Club*

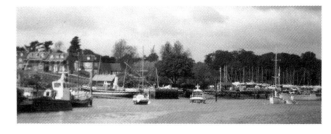

18.4 *The Master Builder pub to the left of Buckler's Hard jetty*

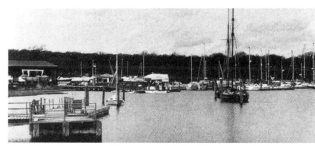

18.5 *Beaulieu Yacht Harbour with Buckler's Hard pier to the left, fuelling pontoon and Harbour Master's office beyond*

from the starboard hand marked by an unlit G buoy (the only one in the river). Observe it.

Anchorage Owing to the large numbers of moorings, yachts may anchor only in the long reach between the prohibited anchorage W of the entrance and Need's Oar Point, as shown on the plan.

There are pile moorings near *Buckler's Hard* to accommodate about 100 visiting yachts; other moorings temporarily vacant can sometimes be had on application to the HM, whose office is at the *Yacht Harbour Marina*. Here there are 100 berths and a yacht yard (tel. 059063–200). He does not keep VHF watch.

Facilities Water and fuel at the Yacht Harbour where there is a boatyard and chandlery. Customs are based there. At Buckler's Hard there are the Master Builder's Hotel, the Maritime Museum and a good village store, with deep freeze,

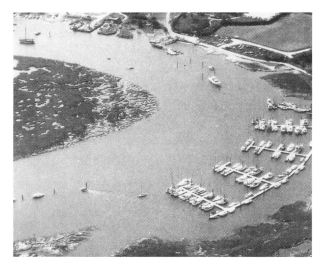

18.6 *Yacht Harbour and Buckler's Hard looking downstream (Aerofilms Ltd)*

which opens every day. There is also a taxi service. Grid-iron and launching site at Buckler's Hard or from beach at Lepe opposite the entrance to the river; both with convenient car parks. Yacht clubs: Beaulieu River SC at Need's Oar Pt and R. Southampton YC at Ginn's Farm. Nearest stations Beaulieu Road, or Brockenhurst 6 miles.

Weather See Southampton p. 129.

*19 Newtown River

Charts: BA 2021; Im 20; Stan 11

Double High Water *First HW Springs approx. −00h. 30m. Dover.*
Heights above Datum *MHWS 3m4. MLWS 0m5. MHWN 2m8. MLWN 1m5.*
Depths *About 0m9 on the bar charted, but more reported (1989) up to 1m8, then 3m3 to Fishhouse Point. Within the harbour from 1m2 to 0m9 as far as Causeway Lake.*

THE HAMLET OF NEWTOWN was once the capital of the Island and vessels of all sizes used the river as a harbour. Romans sacked the town, and then in 1377 it was burnt to the ground by the French. Today only the old town hall and over-grown tracks through the trees, which were once busy streets, recall its importance. But, where once lay fourteenth-century sailing ships, the anchorage is now crowded in weekends during the season. The river, the marshlands and woods retain much of their original character. The National Trust owns the Estuary and much of the adjoining land and marshes which are the nesting places of countless sea birds. Landing at Fishhouse Point is not allowed during the nesting season, April to June.

Approach and Entrance The entrance to Newtown River

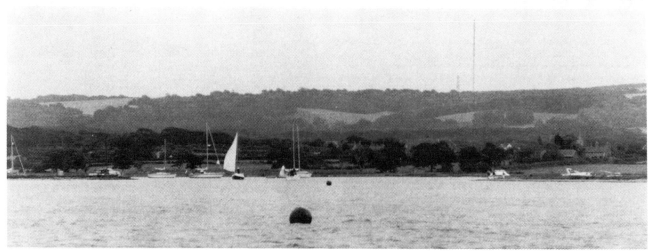

19.1 *Approach on 126° passing between two spherical buoys. Note TV mast on skyline*

is $3\frac{1}{2}$ miles E of Yarmouth and $\frac{3}{4}$ mile eastward of Hamstead Point, which is the most pronounced headland between Yarmouth and Gurnard. It will be identified with certainty when the Hamstead Ledge G con buoy FL (2) G 5s. is sighted. The bar lies $\frac{3}{4}$ mile ESE of this buoy.

Keep near a line joining the Hamstead Ledge buoy with another G con buoy, Salt Mead, until the leading marks are identified. They are inconspicuous and the R porthand buoy marking the 2mo line off the entrance does not have the topmark shown on the charts and is no bigger than a dinghy racing mark. A rough guide is to keep the TV mast on the skyline bearing 147°. The leading marks are on the foreshore on the E side of the entrance. The outer post is RW with a white 'Y' topmark and the inner one a white disc within a black ring. Alter course to 125° on these marks, and allow for a strong current across. Leave the bar buoy (R Sph) to port and the second (G Sph) marking a gravel spit projecting towards the channel, to starboard. When the 'Y' post is close ahead, alter course for the entrance between the shingle points, marked by small R can buoys to port and perches with some G paint to starboard. Here the tide conforms to the direction of the channel.

To starboard there is a shingle spit which is fairly steep-to, but beyond it is mud, while on the port hand a little farther in is another fairly steep shingle point, Fishhouse Point. Beyond this the channel divides; the port hand one is Clamerkin Lake, but the main channel runs in a SSW direction. The NE arm to Clamerkin Lake only has R perches, but there is a G con buoy where the channel swings to the ESE. The SSW arm towards the Causeway lake is marked by R and G perches.

Anchorage The principal anchorage is between the junction of the main channel with Clamerkin Lake (where there is 2m7) and the junction with Causeway Lake $\frac{1}{4}$ mile farther S where there is about 1mo at LW. Private moorings occupy the best positions in about 1m8, so that the visitor will have to

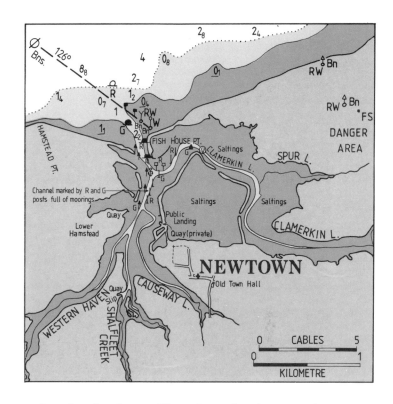

anchor where best he can. The anchorage is rather exposed to NE winds. Alternatively, there is anchorage at the lower end of Clamerkin Lake in 1m2 and rather more water farther up the lake where there are moorings, just above the G con buoy, three of which are for visitors. The holding ground in this vicinity is good. Moorings can sometimes be obtained on application to the HM (tel. 098–378424). Dues help the upkeep of river and moorings; if not collected make a donation in the box beside the boathouse. Smaller craft that can take the mud at LW will find room farther up the main channel. There are no lights on the river or its approaches.

Facilities Water at tap at south end of footbridge and Lower Hamstead farm. Farm produce from farms at Shalfleet or Newtown, but there are no shops at Newtown.

There is a small slip and boatyard at Lower Hamstead and another small yard at Shalfleet Quay. Shalfleet is 2 miles from the anchorage and can be reached by dinghy. There are bus services to Newport and Yarmouth and a small shop and an inn renowned for its clams. Fuel and paraffin at Shalfleet Service Station on main road.

Weather See Southampton p. 129.

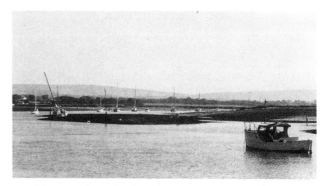

19.2 *Most popular point for going aground is on the west side of the entrance. Western Haven beyond*

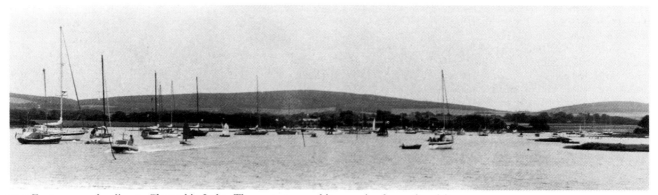

19.3 *Eastern arm leading to Clamerkin Lake. There are some white mooring buoys for visitors*

20 Yarmouth Harbour

Charts: BA 2021; Im Y20; Stan 11

Double High Water *First HW Springs −00h. 51m. Dover.*
Heights above Datum *MHWS 3m1. MLWS 0m6. MHWN 2m5. MLWN 1m4.*
Depths *Tide gauges are placed on the pier facing N for incoming vessels and on the dolphin facing S for vessels leaving the harbour. There is 1m3 in the entrance and from 2m3 to 1m3 within the harbour itself.*

YARMOUTH is a good protected harbour at all states of the tide. The town itself is beautiful, especially viewed from seaward. It is one of the most popular ports on the Solent; yachts have sometimes to be refused entry in summer weekends.

Approach and Entrance Yarmouth can be located from a considerable distance by its conspicuous pier with 2 F R Lts at its end. There is plenty of water in the approaches from E or W off the pierhead, but there is a local tide rip near the Black Rock (marked by an unlit G con buoy) about 4 cables to the westward of Yarmouth pier. With sufficient tide small craft can pass inside the Black Rock (dries 0m8) by keeping the end of the Victoria pier (a cable E of Sconce Point) in line with the S side of Hurst Castle. This passage carries 0m4 but do not go N of the line until Black Rock has been passed.

The harbour entrance lies W of the pier, and there are leading marks, consisting of two posts surmounted by W diamonds with two horizontal B lines each with F G Lt on 187°, which indicate the best water in the approach channel. At the entrance there is a large dolphin (Fl G 5s. 1M) with tide-gauge (used for warping the ferry under bad conditions) close to the end of the breakwater on the starboard hand and the ferry jetty on the port hand

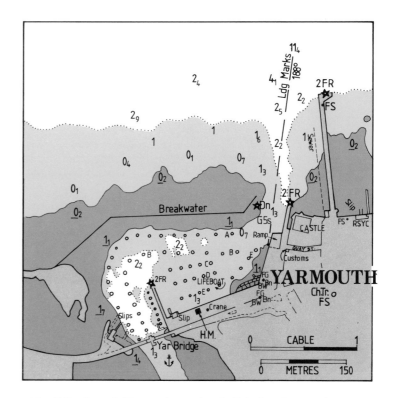

with 2 F R at its end. Keep to the porthand off the jetty but stand out to avoid the slipway at its inner end, then bear to starboard towards the rows of piles. The HM usually gives berthing instructions from a boat, otherwise make contact at his office on the fuelling point on S Quay. The harbour has rows of pile

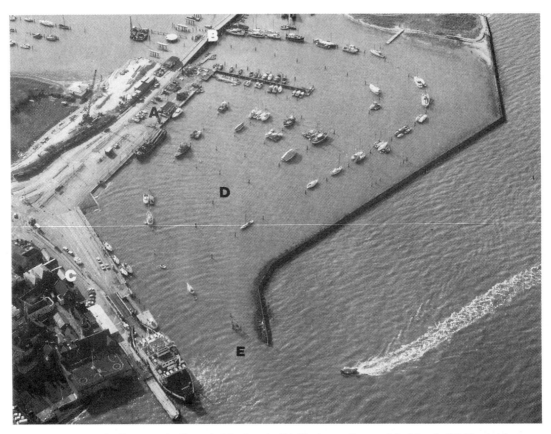

20.1 *Shot of untypically empty harbour (mid-winter). (A) Harbour office and fuel berth (B) Yar bridge and upstream moorings (C) Customs (D) Empty pile moorings (E) Warping dolphin*

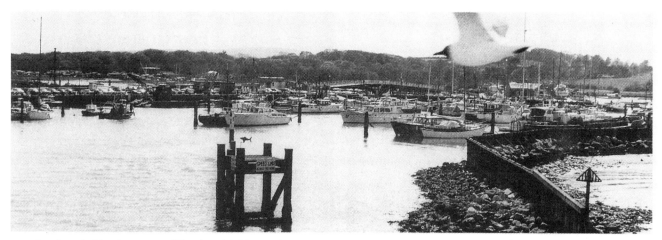

20.2 *Starboard side of entrance. Warping dolphin carries Lt G 5s., tide gauge and warning of 4-knots speed limit*

moorings designated by letters A–E with numbers for each berth, between which are narrow fairways and depths range from 2m2 to 1m3. There is little room for a yacht to tack so use auxiliary power, or warp into position. When the harbour is full a R flag is hoisted at a flagpole at the seaward end of the ferry jetty at the harbour entrance, or at night two R Lts Vert are exhibited from the same point. Yachts may then enter only with permission of the HM. Tel. 0983–760300. No VHF.

Moorings and Anchorage Yachts berth alongside each other, between the mooring piles. The HM will indicate which berth to take. Each line of piles has a letter and each pile a number. It is forbidden to anchor in the harbour, but above the swingbridge (arrange time to open with HM – usually once every 2 h. in daylight) there is some room in which to anchor in the river. Outside anchor to W or E of the end of the pier, although the swell from passing ships causes some discomfort and the anchorage is exposed to northerly winds. Bring up a little inside the line of the pier end if possible.

Facilities There are three yacht yards, marine engineer and scrubbing berths. Good yacht chandler and ironmongery. Water and fuel at New Quay. Customs Office alongside ferry ramp. Yarmouth is a compact little town with hotels and restaurants. Quay St shops include chandler, PO and bookseller. EC Thurs. Dinghy compound. Launching sites from dinghy slips at the Quay or from the ferry slip by arrangement with the HM; car park adjacent. Frequent car ferries to Lymington. Buses to Newport. Yacht club: R. Solent YC.

Weather See Southampton p. 129.

21 Lymington

Charts: BA 2021; Im C3; Stan 11·

Double High Water *First HW Springs —00h. 41m. Dover.*
Heights above Datum *MHWS 3m0. MLWS 0m5. MHWN 2m6. MLWN 1m3.*
Depths *Least depth 2m4 in mid-channel to the Ferry Terminal. Depths then decrease to 0m9 off the Town Quay with a 0m3 shoal a cable short of it.*

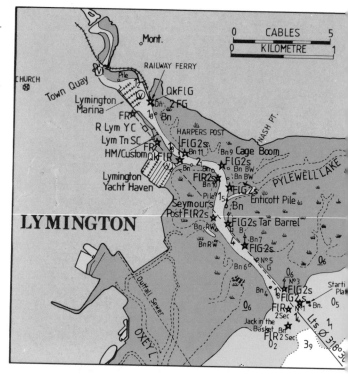

LYMINGTON RIVER is a good harbour for yachts at all states of the tide. The town is charming with excellent facilities of every kind including 750 alongside berths at two marinas and very active yacht clubs which have made it one of the most important racing centres in the Solent. It is the home of several top designers.

Approach and Entrance The entrance lies about 2½ miles NE of Hurst Castle. Whether approaching from W or E keep well away from the extensive shoal water. The first mark which will probably be identified is the starting platform for races on the east side of the entrance. Nearer, the red Jack-in-the-Basket Bn Fl R 2s. on the port hand at the mouth of the river will be seen. The Royal Lymington Clubhouse 1¼ miles up the river is also conspicuous. The two F R leading Lts on course 318½° are situated either side of the Clubhouse on 17 and 12m poles, with 8M visibility. Once the entrance has been identified by passing between No. 1 G buoy (Fl G 2s.) and No. 2 'Cross Boom' buoy (Fl R 2s.), the rest is easy, as the winding channel is clearly marked by R posts with can topmarks to port and G poles with triangular topmarks to starboard. At the first short hitch to starboard, there are separate inward and outward-bound leading marks to enable the ferries to pass each other more easily; one

pair BW N of Enicott Pile (Fl G 2s.) leading 007° for inbound ferries; the other a R pair S of Seymour Post (Fl R 2s.) on course 188°. The car ferries have right of way at all times.

Three cables along the Short Reach there is the entrance to Lymington Yacht Haven opposite No. 11 G pile (Fl G 2s.); there are the two F Y leading lights on 244° to guide you in. The

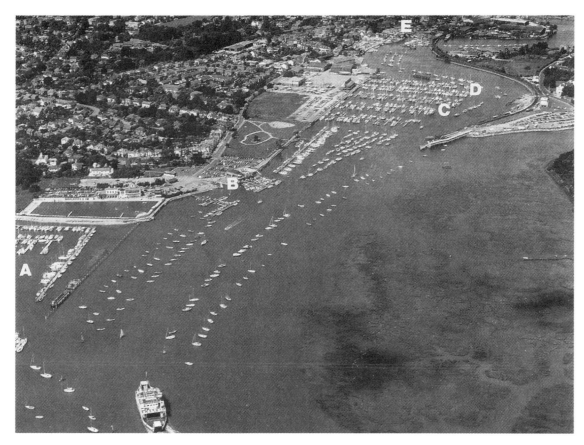

21.1 *(A) Lymington Yacht Haven (B) Royal Lymington Yacht Club (C) Lymington Marina (D) Fuel pontoon (E) Town Quay*

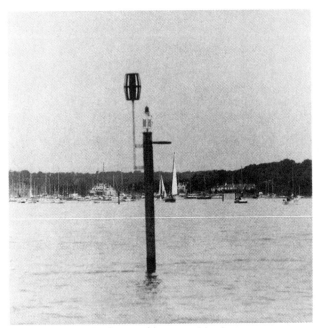

21.2 *Jack-in-the-Basket marking port side of seaward end of the channel*

Anchorage Anchoring is prohibited in the river, which is full of Lymington Harbour Commissioners' moorings. These should not be picked up without permission. Arrangements for berthing, particularly for large yachts, should be made with the HM by telephone (0590–72014). There are berths for upwards of 100 visiting yachts apart from in the marinas, as follows:
(1) *On mooring buoys below the bridge* where there is about 0m9, but a soft bottom so that the keel sinks into the mud and yachts remain upright at low water.
(2) *Alongside Town Quay* just short of the railway bridge, 50m long, up to six abreast with about 1m3 some 6m from the quay, i.e., third berth out.
(3) Berths are often vacant at the marinas, the *Lymington Yacht Haven* in Harper's Lake or the *Lymington Marina* off the Berthon Yard, 100 visitors' berths at each. Contact on VHF Ch 37 or tel. 0590–77071 or 73312 respectively.
(4) Anchoring outside the river is possible in offshore winds and settled weather.

Facilities are outstanding. First-class yacht builders and repairers for all sizes of yachts. Leading international sailmakers for ocean racing and other classes and two smaller sailmakers. Customs. Brooks & Gatehouse electronics. Water at Bath Road pontoon and Town Quay and at marina pontoons where fuel is available. Hotels, restaurants, inns, banks and shops of all kinds. EC Wed. Stations at Ferry Terminal and Town linking with express service from Brockenhurst. Car ferries to Yarmouth. Bus services to all parts. Launching sites at public slipway adjacent yacht club, or at slipway at Town Quay. Car parks near. Yacht clubs: R. Lymington YC, Lymington Town SC.

Weather See Southampton p. 129.

course is now NW'ly past the YC heading for the rail/ferry jetty with 2F at its seaward end. The fairway swings outside the pontoons of the Lymington Marina, past the fuel barge and so to the Town Quay on the W bank. There is shoal water to starboard, so it is necessary to keep well over to port. Even there a 0m3 patch in the fairway may cause some anxiety.

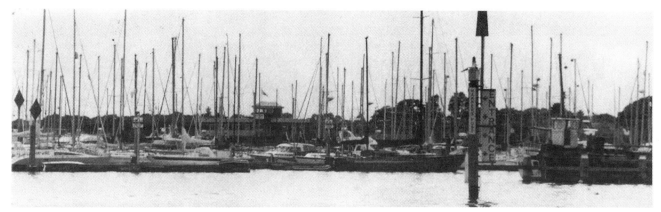

21.3 *Harper's Post Beacon and entrance to Lymington Yacht Haven*

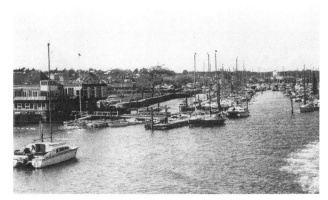

21.4 *Royal Lymington Yacht Club and members' berths*

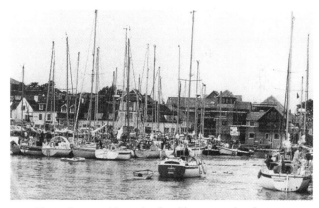

21.5 *Town Quay, with yachts berthing up to six abreast*

*22 Keyhaven

Charts: BA 2021; Im Y20; Stan 11

Double High Water *at Hurst. First HW Springs −ooh. 55m. Dover.*

Heights above Datum *MHWS 2m7. MLWS om5. MHWN 2m3. MLWN 1m3.*

Depths *On the bar om3 but liable to alter. Once inside between 3 and 4m. About 1m5 off Mount Lake, then gradually decreasing to om2 at the quay.*

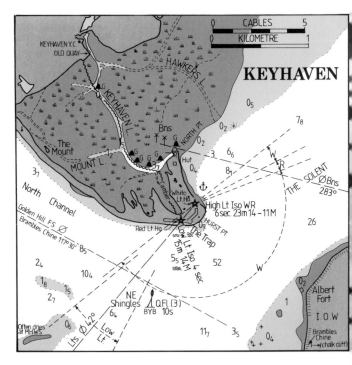

THE ENTRANCE to KEYHAVEN is exposed to easterly winds, but in normal conditions the river makes a very pleasant harbour for small craft. It is so crowded with moorings that there is no room left to anchor except near the entrance. The bar makes the entrance inconvenient; normally accessible at half tide.

Approach and Entrance Keyhaven lies on the north side of the Solent, 4 cables NNW of Hurst Point. If crossing the Solent allow for the strong tidal streams across one's track. It runs S'ly −1 h. to +5 h. HW Dover, max 2½ kts.

The entrance to Keyhaven Lake lies at North Point, the end of the shingle spit extending from Hurst Point. The point is conspicuous and stands out as a low sand and shingle promontory against a background of mud flats. There are two very inconspicuous leading marks on the flats, each with 'X' topmarks on course 283°, but there is only om3 at MLWS. No lights.

Shape a course for a position about ¼ mile NE of the old pier near Hurst High Lt; then approach the entrance at about WNW with Yarmouth open astern. A small G buoy to be left to starboard at the entrance and a R buoy to port, when course must be altered very sharply as North Point comes abeam to leave its steep shingle extremity about 10m to port and the

second of the series of Sph G buoys to starboard. The channel at first bears to SW and is at least 2m deep almost as far as Mount Lake; it is clearly marked by the starboard-hand buoys in the first reach and around the bend to NW as far as Mount Lake. Above that there are one or two porthand R buoys and, 3 cables short of Keyhaven where the channel turns northwards, a G con buoy at the end of Long Reach. The trend of the channel can be

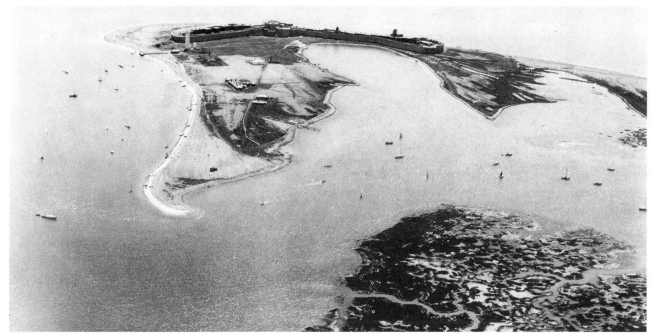

22.1 *Entrance to Keyhaven with Hurst Castle beyond (Brian Manley)*

judged by the line of yachts on moorings in the centre, or farther upstream, where it is very shallow, by a double line of smaller craft. Near HW it is possible to enter through Hawkers Lake keeping close to the line of boat moorings.

Anchorage The only anchorage in the Lake lies between N Point and the first of the private moorings which occupy the whole river farther up. There is a good anchorage in moderate westerly winds off the old pier near Hurst High Lt. To the north of it the water soon begins to shoal so that it becomes necessary to take soundings and anchor farther from the shore. Close to the old pier the anchorage in Hurst Roads is tolerable even in strong SW winds, but good ground tackle is needed as there are

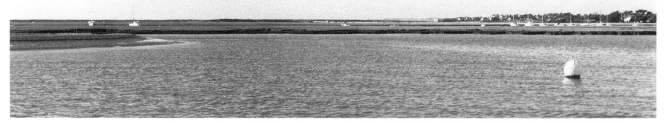

22.2 *Entrance from Solent, with R spherical porthand buoy to the right and North Point to the left*

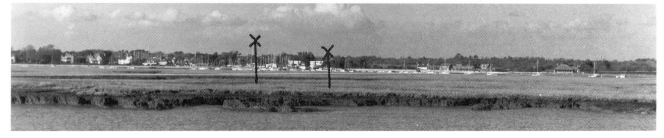

22.3 *Leading marks on 265° here touched up, but in reality inconspicuous*

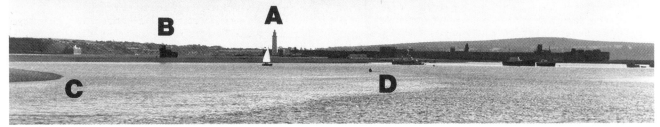

22.4 *(A) Hurst Point High lighthouse (B) Conspicuous watch-hut (C) North Point (D) First of a succession of starboard-hand G spherical buoys*

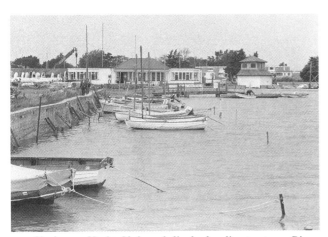

22.5 *Keyhaven Yacht Club and dinghy landing pontoon. River Warden's office in two-storied building to right of YC*

strong tides. Contact River Warden next to YC (tel. 0590–45695) for temporary moorings.

Facilities   Landing steps at the end of Keyhaven Old Quay, at New Quay beyond the yacht club but shallow at LWS. West Solent Boat-builder for repairs and laying up. Hard for scrubbing with 1m8 at MHWS. Water and fuel from boatyard. Hospitable Gun Inn, general stores, PO. EC Thurs. Occasional buses. At Milford-on-Sea, 1 mile, usual facilities of a small seaside town. EC Wed. Launching sites at Keyhaven hards with car park adjacent. Yacht clubs: Hurst Castle SC on N Point; Keyhaven YC at head of the lake is friendly; tel. 0590–42165. No VHF. Ferry Keyhaven–Hurst Castle.

Weather   See Southampton p. 129.

*23   Christchurch

Charts: BA 2219; Im C4; Stan 12

Double High Water *at entrance. First HW Springs −02h. 16m. Dover, which is higher than the Second HW about 3h. later. At Town Quay 2m. after entrance. HW at Neaps is variable, but Second HW is higher and may occur about +02h. 00m. Dover. At Neaps enter between two HWs.*

Heights above Datum *(in harbour) MHWS 1m8. MLWS 0m4. MHWN 1m4. MLWN 0m6.*

Depths   *About 0m1 on bar, but variable and may be lower in prolonged N and NE winds. Off Mudeford Quay about 2m2. In the channel up to Christchurch there is considerable variation in depth – from 0m3 to 2m9.*

OWING to the shallow water over the bar 1m8 is about the maximum draught for entry, except on exceptionally high tides or with local knowledge. But once past the entrance, CHRISTCHURCH harbour is an interesting place to visit. At Mudeford there is good bathing, and Christchurch itself is a beautiful old town, famous for its priory at the junction of the River Avon and River Stour two miles from the entrance.

Approach and Entrance   The entrance to Christchurch lies about a mile N of the conspicuous Hengistbury Head. The bar shifts frequently and varies in depth. Fresh onshore winds between S and E make the entrance dangerous, but in westerly winds some shelter is provided by Hengistbury Head.

There are two dangers when approaching from the west: the Christchurch ledges and Yarranton rocks off the shore of the entrance. From the NE there are no outlying dangers. From N Head buoy at the end of the North Channel or from the seaward end of the Needles Channel head for the right hand edge of

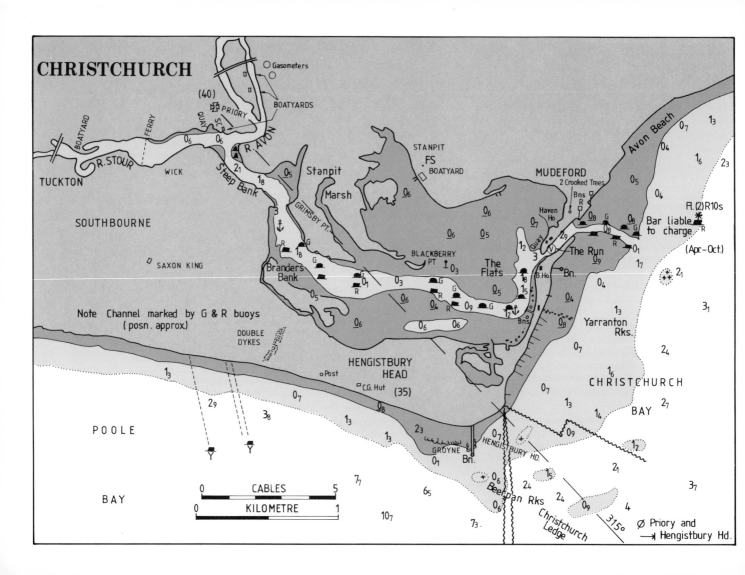

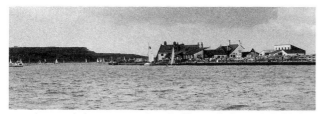

23.1 *Approach from seaward end of buoyed channel. Initial course tends towards right-hand edge of Mudeford Haven Quay*

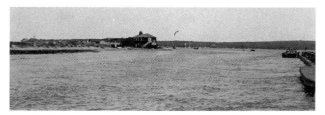

23.2 *The Run with Hengistbury Head beyond yachts at anchor inside*

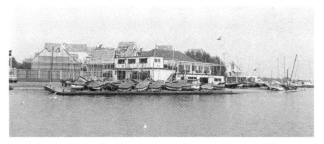

23.3 *Christchurch Sailing Club from the entrance to River Stour, with new property development all around it*

Hengistbury Head, keeping Christchurch Priory tower well open to its right. The channel across the bar in 0m4 is very shallow, narrow and varies in position and depths, so arrive on a rising tide or wait at anchor outside the 2m0 line. The channel is marked by buoys, R to port and G to starboard, but these may drag after gales. There are two landmarks which assist: Haven House at the quay on the far side of the entrance bearing about 260° and a conspicuous big house near the beach among trees opposite the outer pair of buoys. Once the outer buoys have been identified, the channel may be entered. At the innermost R buoy the channel bends sharply to port leaving the sea wall and the quay to starboard and the spit of submerged land to port. This channel is 'The Run', where there is 3–5 kts tidal stream, up to 9 kts on an exceptional spring ebb, but a depth of at least 2m0 at the quay.

Continuing up to Christchurch, the channel is well marked by small R buoys to port and G to starboard. The streams are much weaker but the depth is lower to the east of Branders Bank than it is on the bar. Finally head for the Priory with the SC flagstaff in front of it. Speed limit 5 kts.

Moorings and Anchorage Christchurch Harbour is full of moorings. Enquire at Quay & Moorings Supt (04252–4933), at

Christchurch SC; they have two visitors' moorings or Christchurch Marine, tel. 0202–483250, keep two deepwater moorings available. Yachts can anchor anywhere that room can be found but keep clear of the centre of the buoyed channel and avoid anchoring in The Run. Multi-hulls and twin-keelers can dry out off the fairway.

Facilities Three yacht yards. Water and fuel at Christchurch Marine jetty. Hotel, restaurants, banks, PO and many shops (EC Wed.) at Christchurch. Launching sites:

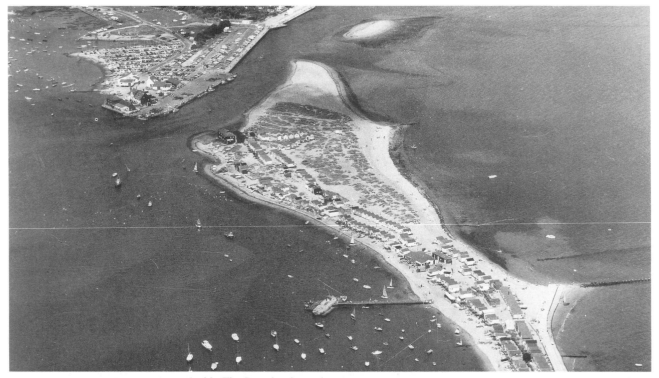

23.4 *Shifting sands off the entrance. Inside The Run the channel runs past the pier and then swings clockwise towards Christchurch*

(1) Slipway at Christchurch Quay.
(2) At sailing club, by permission.
(3) At yacht yard.
(4) From beach on harbour side of Mudeford Haven Quay. Car parks near by. Frequent buses and local trains from Christchurch. Airport at Hurn. Yacht Clubs: Christchurch SC and Highcliffe SC.

Weather   See Southampton p. 129.

24 Poole Harbour

Charts: BA 2611; Im Y23; Stan 12

High Water *There are double tides in Poole Harbour. At entrance first HW Springs −02h. 36m. Dover, with second HW 3h. later, but only 0m5 lower. Town quay has first HW Springs 2h. before Dover. At Neaps these occur 5h. and 4½h. before Dover, but range is small – indeed second HW Neaps is fractionally higher than first, amounting to a lengthy stand at HW.*

HW at Wareham is about 1h. later than at Pool Quay.

Heights above datum

	MHWS	MLWS	MHWN	MLWN
Entrance	2m0	0m3	1m6	1m1
Town Quay	2m2	0m4	1m8	1m2
Wareham	2m2	0m7	1m7	1m1

Depths *From the Bar buoy (No. 1) as far as Town Quay the Swash and Middle Ship Channels are dredged to a least depth of 5m0. The Old Main Channel past Salterns Marina has 3m6. Other depths as on chart.*

POOLE's importance both as a commercial and yacht harbour has been greatly enhanced since the new 5m0 channel has been dredged along the former Diver Channel, leading to alongside and RO/RO berths at Lower Hamworthy and a new sheltered 350-berth marina and clubhouse for Poole YC as part of the development. It must be one of the finest in Britain.

Approach and Entrance The prominent feature in the approach to Poole is the chalk Handfast Pt, with Old Harry Rocks off it. The new Fairway buoy (safewater RW Fl 10s.) is 6½ cables NE of the Pt. The Bar buoy is situated a mile north-north-east of it; about 2 miles beyond the buoy will be seen the harbour entrance, with the conspicuous Haven Hotel on the east side.

During the ebb there is a tide-rip off Handfast Pt. Strong winds between E and S can kick up a nasty chop in the Swash while the ebb is running.

The Swash Channel runs 335° from between the Bar buoy

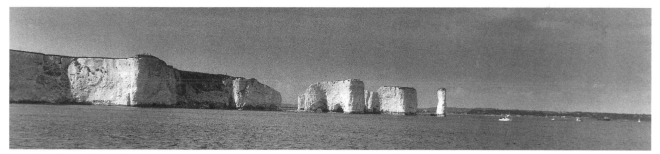

24.1 *Old Harry (Handfast Point) three-quarters of a mile south-west of the Fairway buoy. As conspicuous as the Needles*

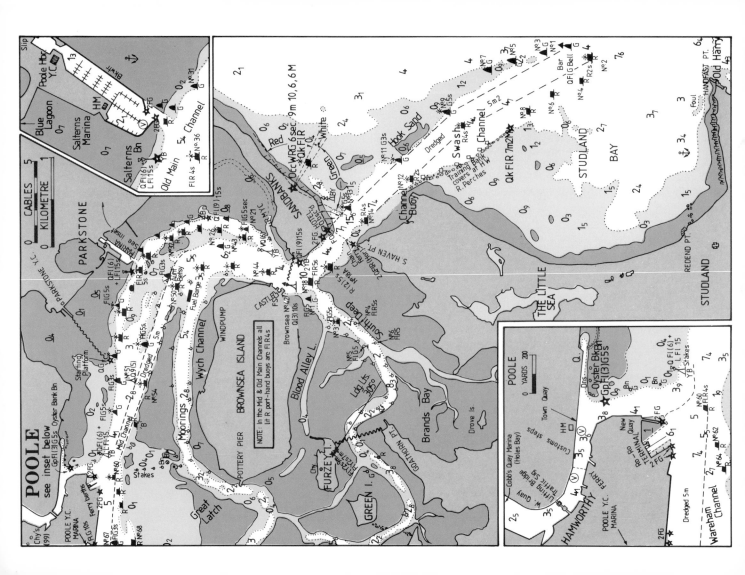

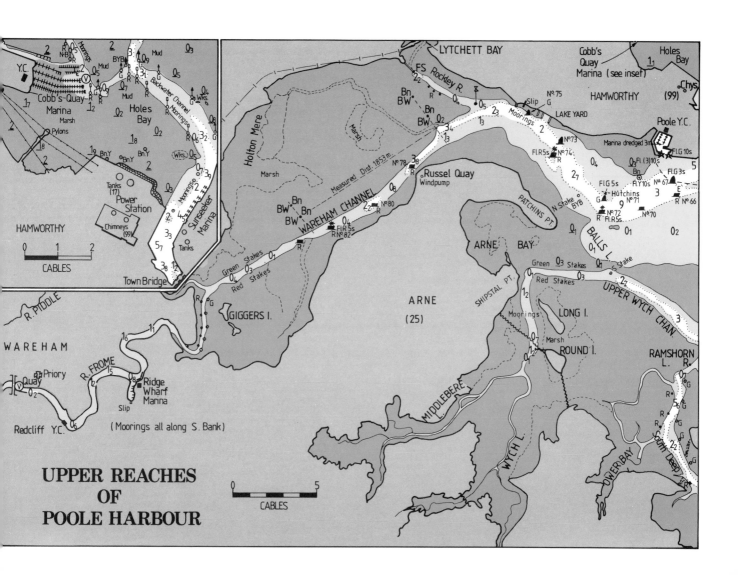

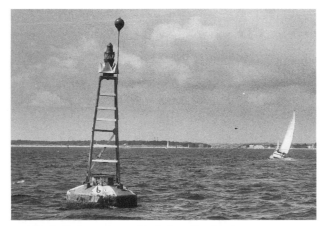

24.2 *Poole Fairway buoy. Yacht heading for the entrance on 330°*

(No. 1 G con Q G Bell) and No. 2 R can (R 2s.). There are unlit buoys on either side (Nos. 3–8) before leaving to port the R Dolphin at the seaward end of the Training Bank (Q R 7m. 2M); 700yds farther the channel passes between No. 9 G con (G 5s.) at the NE end of Hook Sand and No. 12 R can (R 2s.). The course is then 320° until the narrows with No. 13 G con (G 5s.) and No. 14 R can (R 4s.) on either side. Leave the conspicuous Haven Hotel to starboard and watch out for the chain ferry.

Inside the entrance the channel divides. One arm (South Deep) runs SW while the main channel to Poole swings round between Sandbanks and Brownsea Is. in a NNE direction.

East Looe This channel is a short cut off Sandbanks if arriving from the direction of Bournemouth. Head for No. 16A buoy (Q R) 2 cables offshore and about ½ mile NE of the entrance. It is not recommended at night, but, if you must,

approach in the W sector of the E Looe Lt. (Oc G 6 WRG 9m 10M) and leave it close to port. Then steer 245° to about 100m off Sandbanks Hotel, where you join the Swash channel, leaving the ends of the groynes to starboard and No. 13 G con Swashway buoy clear to port. The least water is 1m8 ESE from No. 16 A buoy.

Harbour channels Head from the entrance towards the E-cardinal Brownsea buoy (G (3) 10s.), thence altering to the NNE towards the S-cardinal S Middle No. 20 buoy (VQ (6) +LFl 15s.) which marks the point where the two principal channels towards Poole Town divide.

The Middle Ship Channel is now dredged to 5m0 and is the most direct if heading for the Town or beyond. Leave No. 20 S-cardinal buoy (Q(6) + LFl 15s.) to starboard by altering to N so as to pass between No. 43 G con (G 3s.) and No. 46 R can (R 4s.). The channel is now well marked by a succession of numbered buoys, each with same characteristics as the two above, although not all of them are lit. A slow swing to port up to No. 50 R 'Aunt Betty' buoy enters the 1.2 mile straight fairway on course 290° up to the S-cardinal Stakes buoy No. 55 (Q (6) +LFl 15s.), where you either head 343° up the Little Channel to Town Quay and beyond, or alter to port to 273° parallel with the commercial docks for Poole YC Marina or to pick up the Wareham Channel and the R. Frome. Yachts must give way to commercial traffic; in places along the Middle Ship Channel there is little room to do so, but it is not impossible.

The Old Main Channel leads to the Salterns Marina complex or Parkstone Lake. Leave No. 20 S Middle buoy to port on 035° to pass between No. 22 R can (R 4s.) and no. 21 'Jack Jones' G con buoy (G 5s.). The channel is clearly marked, with most buoys lit R 4s. or G 5s. Take a slow swing through N to 325° until No. 36 Salterns R buoy is broad on the port bow, with the S-cardinal Salterns Bn (Q (6) +LfL 15s.) right ahead. At this point the W pierhead of Salterns Marina (2F R) will be

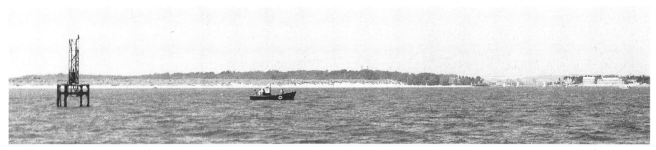

24.3 Beacon at seaward end of the training wall on west side of Swash Channel

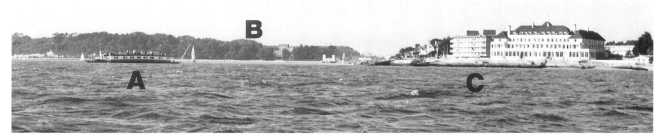

24.4 (A) Chain ferry (B) Brownsea Island (C) Sandbanks Hotel

abeam. Go for it, passing between unlit R and G buoys to swing hard to port and enter, leaving the E pierhead (2F G) on the starboard hand. If going farther up the channel, leave Salterns Bn to starboard and follow the marked channel, finally on 265° to join the Middle Ship Channel near its NW end, with No. 41 G (Fl G 5s.) close to starboard.

The Wych Channel starts near the fuel barge close to No. 48 buoy and runs close parallel to the N shore of Brownsea Is. between unlit R and G posts with topmarks. There is an E-cardinal post where the channel heads due N as Wills Cut until it joins the Little Channel for the Town.

South Deep runs SW from No. 18 R can (R 5s.) opposite N Haven, clearly marked as far as the yacht moorings a mile upstream off Goathorn Pt. Several of the starboard-hand G posts are now lit for the benefit of traffic serving the oil rigs on Furzey Is., which has its own leading marks 305° Fl Y 2s. beyond three buoys (G 5s.) marking the channel close to the landing-point.

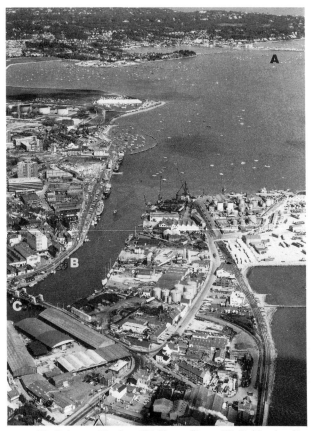

24.5 *(A) Salterns Marina (B) Town Quay (C) Bridge leading to Cobb's Quay Marina*

Wareham channel starts off Lake Pier and the Dorset Yacht yard a mile beyond the commercial docks and Poole YC on the same bank. It has only four R can buoys to mark the $1\frac{1}{2}$ mile straight channel on about 240° until posts take over all the way up to Wareham (R with can topmarks to port; G with triangles to starboard). It shoals quickly to 0m4 where the posts start, so you must read the tides carefully or take advice. Remember, even at LW Neaps there is a bonus of over 1m0. Once in the river, there are yachts moored along its left bank all the way to the bridge at Wareham. The best water is close to them.

Holes Bay Access is through the Town bridge, which opens every 2 h. at weekends from 07.30 to 21.30. Weekday openings are between 09.30 and 23.30. Light signals displayed: R – bridge shut; G – bridge open; RY – open for traffic from the side on which the lights are showing.

Keep to the E bank close past the Sunseeker Marina until reaching the Backwater Channel leading NW between R and G posts with topmarks for 3 cables. At an E-cardinal post (BYB) the channel takes a 90° turn to port, leading straight into Cobb's Quay Marina. There is 2m5 as far as the end of Backwater Channel, after which there is a least depth of 0m1 at MLWS.

Anchorages and Berths

(1) Outside. There is excellent holding ground in *Studland Bay*, protected from westerly and SW winds. Small village with hotels, PO and grocer about $\frac{1}{4}$ mile inshore. EC Thurs.

(2) *Off Brownsea Is.* most of the area is occupied by private moorings. Hail the launchman for advice or enquire at the R. Motor YC or at one of the yacht yards.

(3) Moorings may sometimes be had inside the entrance on the E side in the *North Haven Lake*, off the yacht yard. Apply to boatman, yacht yard or yacht club.

(4) *Poole Harbour YC Marina* at Salterns (240 berths). Turn off to starboard for it at No. 36 R can buoy (Fl R 5s.). The guaranteed dredged depth is 1m5, but there are berths available

for boats up to 2m3. Call the Dock Master from the reception berth just inside the entrance. Call on Ch 37. Tel. 0202–707321.

(5) *Alongside Town Quay* north side (100 berths in trots). The HM is in the main Poole Harbour offices (tel. 0202–685261) but he also has a berthing office in a hut at the quayside. Ch 16 or 14.

(6) *Cobb's Quay Marina* has 1,000 berths. Depths 1m2 at MLWS, 1m8 at MLWN, but soft mud allows deeper draughts. Normal access ±4hrs. HW. Call on Ch 37 callsign 'CQ4' or tel. 0202–674299. Facilities include a dogs' loo.

(7) *Above Poole* off the Dorset Lake Shipyard in Wareham channel, where there are sometimes moorings for hire, and attendance.

(8) *In W arm of harbour*, i.e. in South Deep, as far up as a cable beyond Goathorn Point.

(9) *Poole YC Marina* is strictly private, sometimes available by prior enquiry on tel. 0202–672687. It has 350 pontoon berths with 9ft (2m75) draught, but will not accommodate boats over

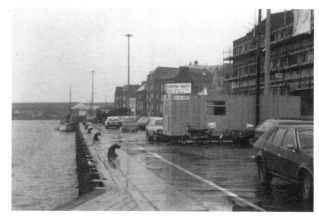

24.6 *Piermaster's office on Town Quay*

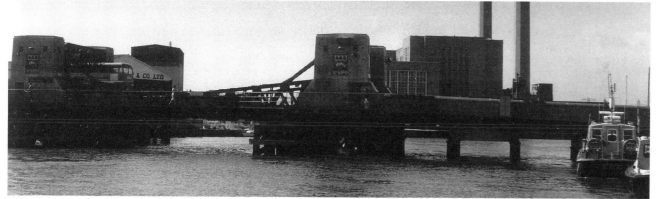

24.7 *Poole Bridge. Hamworthy power station chimneys (conspicuous) upstream on port bank*

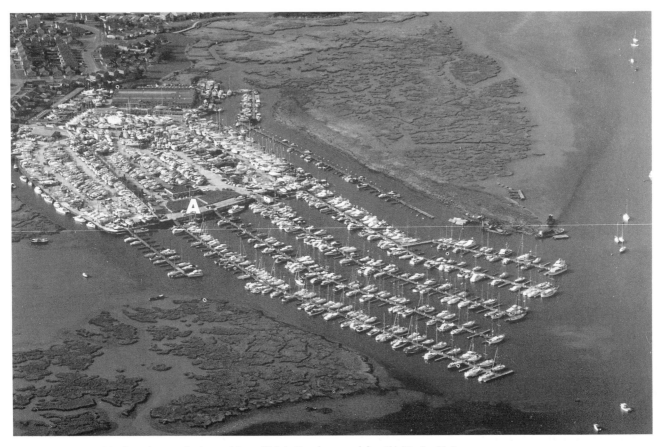

24.8 *Cobb's Quay Marina. Approach channel from Hole's Bay bottom right. (A) Yacht Club*

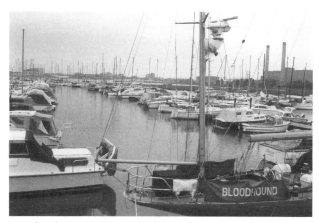

24.9 *Berth nearest Yacht Club has enough water for 'Bloodhound'*

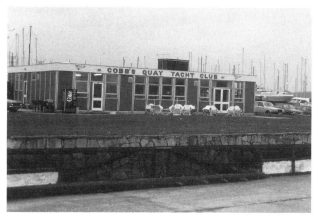

24.10 *Cobb's Quay Yacht Club*

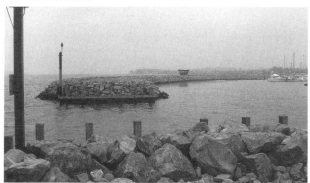

24.11 *Entrance to Poole Yacht Club Marina. Race Committee hut on west arm of breakwater*

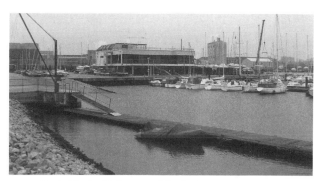

24.12 *Poole Yacht Club – possibly the best appointed clubhouse and yacht harbour in England. Restricted to boats less than 40ft LOA belonging to members*

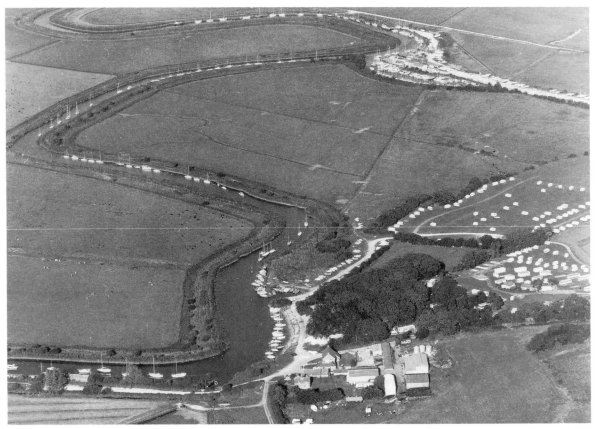

24.13 *River Frome facing downstream from the last bend before Wareham. Redcliffe Yacht Club bottom centre with Ridge Wharf Marina top right. Note boats secured fore-and-aft along left bank*

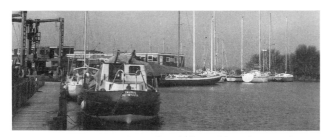

24.14 *Ridge Wharf Marina with 'Galway Blazer' secured alongside marina offices and chandlery*

40ft LOA (12m5). All clubhouse facilities, but a taxi-ride to the nearest shops.

(10) *River Frome.* 170 pontoon berths or moorings either side of Ridge Wharf yacht centre available by arrangement, tel. 09295–2650. Situated in open countryside, but useful for repairs or winter storage. Some berths at Redcliffe YC a little farther upstream. Shallow berths alongside Town Quay just short of road bridge in Wareham. Picturesque, but 0m2 at MLWS. Contact Wessex water authority c/o Old Granary. Tel. 09295–3444.

Anchorage may be found anywhere in Poole Harbour by choosing a position protected from the wind and free from moorings which are laid in all the best spots. In strong winds anchorage in open water areas may be uncomfortable for small craft, but shelter may be found at Poole Quay, or under a weather shore such as the Wych channel (protected from S by Brownsea Is.) or off Goathorn Pt (protection from W and SW). For fuller information call Poole HM on Ch 16.

Facilities Yacht yards at Sandbanks, Parkstone, Cobb's Quay and Hamworthy. Customs office. Water at tap or by hose on application at HM's office at Poole. Petrol at garages at bridge and quay where it is also available alongside in sealed cans or

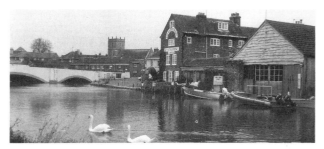

24.15 *Wareham. Public landing on starboard hand just short of bridge*

from all yacht yards and marinas. A refuelling barge is moored in Wych channel near No. 48 buoy. Diesel fuel in bulk from road tankers at Town Quay by arrangement. Ship chandlers. Yacht brokers. Sailmakers. Hotels and many shops. EC Wed. Launching sites: Lilliput Yacht Service, Sandbanks Rd: end of quay farthest from Poole Bridge by arrangement with the crane hirers. Public launching slip at Baiter, E. of Fisherman's Dock. Yacht clubs: Lilliput SC, R. Motor YC, Parkstone YC, Poole Harbour YC, Poole YC, Wareham SC, Redcliffe SC, East Dorset SC, Converted Cruiser Club. Poole Quay YC at Town Quay.

Weather BBC Shipping 1515m LW (198kHz) 0033, 0555, 1355, 1750. Area Wight.

Bournemouth Two Counties Rdo 828kHz (362m.) On the hour. Sea conditions 0708, 0808, 0908, 1306, 1700. Inshore: Fri 1708. Sat 0750, 1310. Sun 0830.

Marinecall. 0898–500457.

Niton Rdo Ch 28, or 1834kHz at 0833, 2033.

Southampton Weather Centre, tel. 0703–228844.

*25   Swanage

Charts: BA 2172; Im 4; Stan 15

Depths   *Over 2mo to within 1 cable of the Bay shore.*

IN SETTLED weather and with winds between WNW and SW there is a pleasant anchorage off the pier (2 F R 6m 3M). When approaching care should be taken to avoid Peveril ledges off the S extremity of Swanage Bay. The tide sets strongly across them. There is an R can buoy 4 cables off the Pt marking the end of the ledges where there is a tidal race particularly on the SSW stream when the wind is contrary and it can be very rough. See Passage Data. Tide 3 kts at Springs, turns NE at +05.30 Dover and to SW at −00.30 Dover.

The anchorage is a cable WNW of the end of the pier in about 2mo, seaward of local moorings, with larger yachts farther out, but the holding ground has weed in parts and is not so good as at Studland Bay, which has the additional advantage of Poole near at hand as a port of refuge in case of a change of wind or weather. Contact Piermaster on 0829–423565.

Excellent hotels and shopping facilities. EC Thurs. Good sailing club (Swanage SC), tel. 0829–422987. Launching site at slipway near pier with car park adjacent. Buses.

Weather   See Poole p. 161.

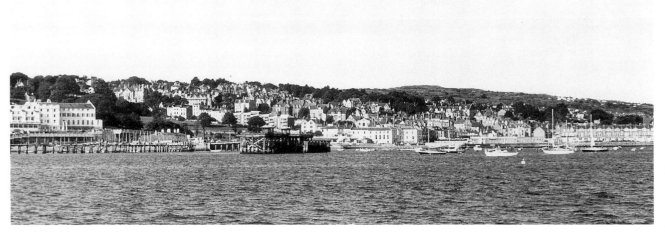

25.1 *Pier in centre, yacht anchorage to the right*

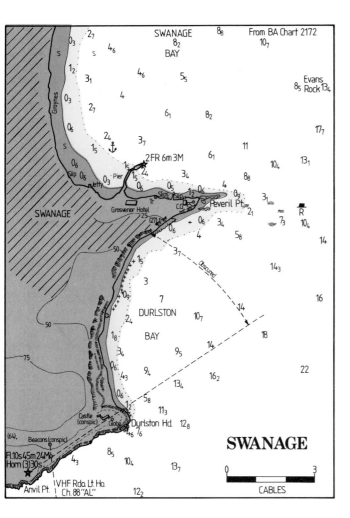

*26 Lulworth Cove

Charts: Im C4; Stan 12

High Water *approx. −04h. 49m. Dover.*
Heights above Datum *MHWS 2m1. MLWS 0m2. MHWN 1m4. MLWN 0m7.*
Depths *About 5m0 in entrance; 3m0 in centre, shallows within 100m of the beach.*

LULWORTH COVE is a famous beauty spot and worth a diversion. There are good walks to the westward, but E of the cove there are gunnery ranges. Red flags are flown when firing is scheduled.

Lulworth should be visited only in settled weather and during offshore winds. A shift of wind to S or SW, bringing with it a strong blow, as so frequently happens, will send a heavy swell into the cove. In such conditions power vessels, let alone yachts, may find it difficult to get out in safety. Therefore, clear out if the weather threatens to change. If caught inside, apply to local boatmen for heavy anchors and cables.

Lulworth Gunnery Ranges There are two danger areas for shipping to the south of Lulworth and Kimmeridge. The one normally in use extends 5M out to sea and the outer, which is seldom used, extends out to 12M. Times of firing are published in local papers and notified to neighbouring HMs and yacht clubs who can supply leaflets giving the details. They can also be obtained from the Range Office, tel. 0929–462721 ext. 819 or 824. When firing is in progress R flags and flag 'U' are flown by day and Lts Fl R shown at night at the huts immediately east of the cove on the summit of Bindon Hill and on St Alban's Head. Vessels may pass through the areas but passage must be made as quickly as possible and anchoring,

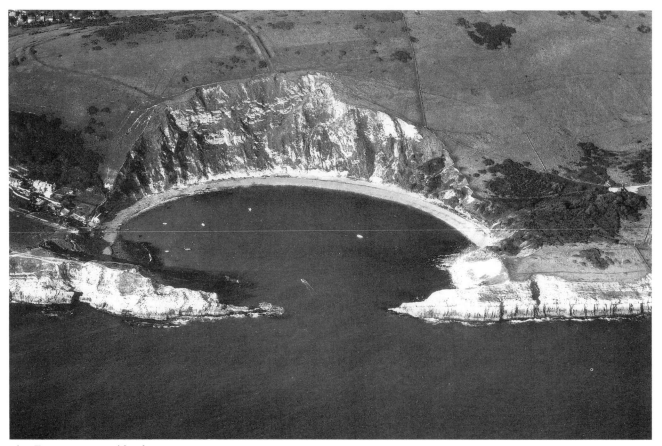

26.1 *Favour eastern side of entrance*

fishing or stopping is prohibited. When the range is active, fast patrol boats are on station to keep yachtsmen clear of the area. Set watch on Ch 8 during firings. Portland Naval Base give firing times on Ch 13 or 14 at 0945 and 1645. Long-range firings rare in August.

Approach and Entrance Lulworth is not always easy to identify from seaward. To the W there runs a series of W cliffs with curved summits. The entrance is just to the E of a sugar-loaf hill with an ex-coastguard hut situated upon it.

There are rocks on both sides of the entrance of the cove but those on the W extend farther than those on the E, so keep slightly E of the centre. Once past these rocks the fairway opens into the wide cove itself.

As may be expected, the wind is fluky or squally at the entrance, and often baffling when entering under sail.

Anchorage No anchorage outside. Anchor in about 2m4 on the N side of the cove where the holding ground is Bu clay or on NW in SW winds. Avoid anchoring in the fairway near the beach landing of Lulworth village on the NW side of cove.

Facilities Water at tap in car park or the beach café may oblige. Petrol and oil at garage. Small hotels, PO. Shops, EC Wed, Sat. Launching site from beach at end of road, with car park adjacent. Provisions at Boon's stores during summer months. Frequent buses in summer months.

Weather See Weymouth p. 169.
BBC forecast area: Portland.
Local forecasts Weymouth Bay. VHF Ch 5 at 0833 and 2033.

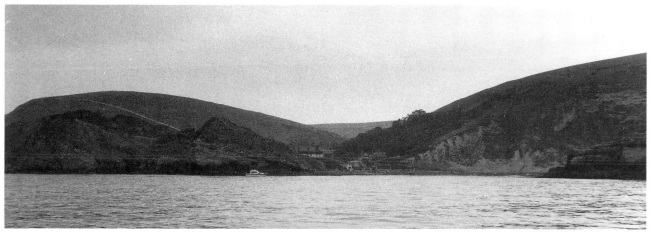

26.2 *View from the south-east. Lulworth village in the centre*

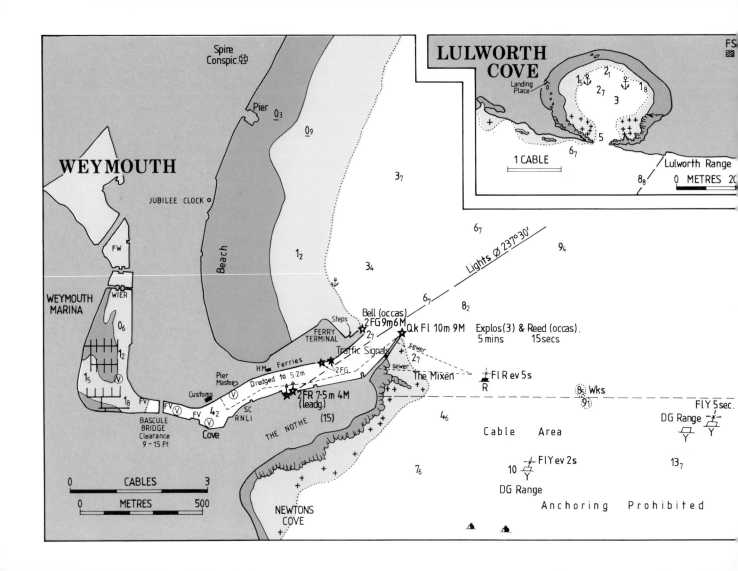

LULWORTH COVE

FS

Landing Place

2_1
1_5
2_7
1_8
3
5
6_7
8_8

Lulworth Range

1 CABLE

0 METRES 20

Spire Conspic.

Pier 0_3

0_9

WEYMOUTH

JUBILEE CLOCK

Beach

3_7

1_2

3_4

6_7

FW

WEYMOUTH MARINA

WIER

0_6

1_2

1_5

1_8 FV

FV

Steps

FERRY TERMINAL

Bell (occas)
2FG 9m 6M

2_7

Traffic Signals

Qk Fl 10m 9M

Explos(3) & Reed (occas).
5 mins   15secs

HM Ferries

Pier Master

Dredged to 5·2m

2FG

sewer

2_7

sewer

The Mixen

Fl R ev 5s
R

Customs

SC
RNLI

4_2

2FR 7·5m 4M
(leadg.)

(15)

THE NOTHE

Cove

FV

FV

8_2

Lights Ø 237°30'

9_4

6_7

8_5 Wks
9_1

FlY 5 sec.

DG Range

Cable   Area

4_6

13_7

7_6

FlY ev 2s
Y

DG Range

10

BASCULE BRIDGE
Clearance
9 - 15 Ft.

Anchoring   Prohibited

CABLES
0   3

METRES
0   500

NEWTONS
COVE

27 Weymouth

Charts: BA 2255, 2268; Im C4; Stan 12

High Water *−04h. 38m. Dover.*
Heights above Datum *MHWS 2m1. MLWS 0m2. MHWN 1m4. MLWN 0m7.*
Tides *The tides are 4 hours flood, 4 hours ebb, and 4 slack subject to the 'Gulder' as it is called, which is a small flood with a rise of approx. 0m2 making its way into the harbour about ¾h. after the first LW.*
Depths *The entrance, and N side, where ships berth is dredged to 5m4. There is less water on the S side.*

WEYMOUTH is a popular seaside resort with many historic buildings along its quaysides. The harbour is sheltered but in strong easterly winds the approach can be rough and there is sometimes an uncomfortable swell in the area of the pierheads.

Approach and Entrance The harbour lies about ½ mile north of the Portland Harbour breakwaters. The entrance is between two piers. On the S is the Nothe Hill, and on the N pier is the Pavilion. The Jubilee Clock – conspicuous – is about ½ mile N along the front. Approaching from the eastward a good transit is by bringing into line the two pierheads on 273°. Several buoys will be seen and should be left well to port. Three of these are light buoys; the outer three are Y (Fl Y ev 5s., Fl Y ev 10s. and Fl Y ev 2s.) degaussing (DG) Range buoys. The closest inshore, off the Mixen rocks, marking the sewer outfall, is a R can (Fl R ev 5s.). Then steer a cable off the entrance and round in between the two piers. The N pier is 2F G 9m 6M with an Occas bell in fog. S pier is Q 10m 9M using explosives ev 5m. in fog and a reed ev. 15s. There are two W triangular leading marks at 237½° on the S quay (each 2F R 7.5m 4M) for ships but they need not be followed by yachts. Keep clear of the fairway in the outer part of the harbour when there are hauling-off warps across the harbour when a cross-Channel ferry is about to depart.

Regulating Signals are displayed by lights on a mast on S Pier:

RRR flashing	Port closed – serious emergency
RRG	Entrance foul – no movement allowed
RRR	No entry allowed – ship sailing
GGG	No departure allowed – ship entering
GWG	Move as directed by HM

When no signals are shown yachts may move at discretion. Storm cones hoisted on mast at N pierhead.

Berthing Visiting yachts may be hailed from the starboard side of the entrance or can contact the Piermaster's office on Ch 16 or 12 and will usually be directed to a berth in the Cove. If the Piermaster's office is not manned (tel. 0305–760276) try the HM by telephone on 0305–760620 or go right up the harbour and moor *alongside the Cove Quay* on the port side about a cable short of the bridge. This is the most popular berth for small yachts. Anchorage outside the harbour may be found in settled weather and offshore winds in 2 to 3m about a cable NW of the end of the pier, clear of the entrance and the turning space required by ferries. Shallow water extends a long way seaward. The depths of water alongside the Cove Quay wall vary from 0m1 to 0m4 at LAT, but a pontoon is usually positioned at the shallowest part. At a distance of 3m off the quay there is 1m0 increasing to 4m towards mid-channel. To the west of the Bascule bridge lies the 580-berth *Weymouth Town Marina*, mostly for small craft, but those with draughts up to 1m8 can lie afloat. Contact by tel. 03057–73538. The clearance under the bridge varies from 9–15 ft as shown on the tide-gauge. Enquire locally about opening times.

Facilities Yacht yards and chandlers. Customs Office.

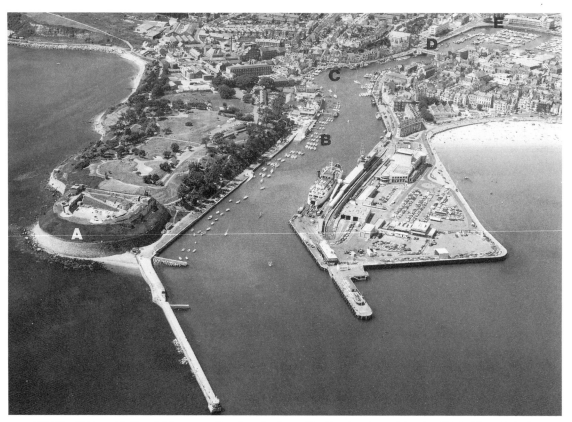

27.1 *(A) The Nothe with South Pier extending from its base. Traffic signals on this pier.(B) Sailing Club (C) The Cove – visitors' berths alongside the wall, with Harbour Office and Customs on right bank (D) Bascule Bridge leading to Weymouth Town Marina at (E)*

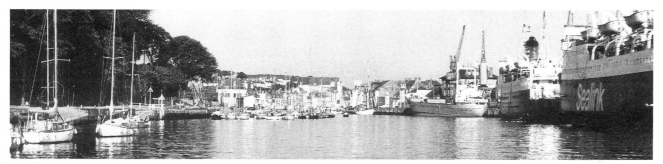

27.2 *Berths for commercial traffic on right. Note leading marks low on left bank, downstream of Sailing Club*

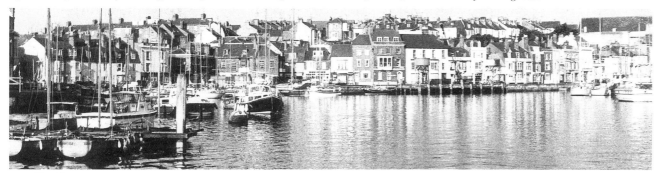

27.3 *The Cove*

Showers and WCs at Piermaster's Office 13 Customs House Quay (N side). Water at cove and at quays. Fuel at quayside, by arrangement. Hotels, restaurants, and shops. EC Wed. Mainline station – with trains to London and Southampton – and buses. Launching sites from slipway in harbour by prior permission of HM or at yards. Yacht clubs: R. Dorset YC, Weymouth SC.

Weather BBC forecast area: Portland.
 VHF Ch 5. Weymouth Bay at 0833, 2033.
 Marinecall tel. 0898–500457.

28 Portland Harbour

Charts: BA 2255, 2268; Im 4; Stan 12

High Water *0.4h. 38m. Dover.*
Heights above Datum *MHWS 2m1. MLWS 0m2. MHWN 1m4. MLWN 0m7.*
Depths *Deep ship harbour except on its western side.*

PORTLAND HARBOUR lies in the bay formed by the mainland to the N, the long narrow strip of the Chesil Beach (mostly pebbles) to the W, and the high peninsula of Portland to the S. From the E it is protected by three big breakwaters built mainly by Napoleonic POWs which create a 3 sq mile artificial harbour. This is primarily a naval base but it also provides shelter for yachts, though it can be uncomfortable in gales or windshifts. Within the harbour there are numerous unlit floating targets, mooring buoys, etc., and chains on the bottom. Frequent naval exercises are carried out from Portland and its adjacent waters with submarines, helicopters and surface craft. Night exercises involve flares and gunfire. The schedules are broadcast on Ch 14 at 0945 and 1645 daily.

Approach and Entrance Portland is easy to identify. It is a high wedge-shaped peninsula that, viewed from seaward, resembles an island. Its highest point (the Verne 44m) is at the northern end; the southern extremity (the Bill) is low, with its conspic. 43m W Lt Ho with R band (Fl (4) 20s. 29M) over the sector 244°–117°. As it sweeps nearer the shore, it cuts to Fl (3) then all the way down to a single flash before it is obscured (141°–S–221°). In fog a dia sounds ev 30s.

The principal danger to navigation in the approach to Portland is the Race. This is the most dangerous disturbance on the whole of the S Coast, and the time of tide has to be studied, but it does not affect yachts approaching from the eastward, who have to watch for the Shambles bank, covered by a F R from the Bill ±10° on 281°.

The harbour itself may be located behind its long stone breakwaters, northward of the heights of Portland. There are only two entrances in use: The E and N Ship channels. The E one has Q R 14m 5M and Fl 10s. 22m 20M to mark the entrance; the other Oc R 15s. 11m 5M and Oc G 10s. 11m 5M as port- and starboard-hand lights. Seek permission to enter on Ch 13 (Q HM or Ops). His tel. 0305–820311.

Regulations Speed limit is 12 knots. Yachts should not approach HM ships or jetties closely and must give way to large power-driven vessels inside the harbour or its entrance.

Anchorage There is anchorage off *Old Castle Cove* in the NW of the harbour, with depths of 2 to 3m. Yachts should anchor outside the yachts on private moorings, of which there are many. It is better if possible to get use of a vacant mooring. Enquire of the boatman or the Castle Cove SC (tel. 0305–783708) at the top of a long steep path. Visiting yachtsmen are usually permitted to use the landing-stage belonging to the sailing club. There is water from a tap on the shore. PO, shops and town are ¼ mile distant. To Weymouth is a walk of over ½ mile or go by bus.

In strong southerly and SW winds this anchorage is too exposed. In this case bring up in the anchorage *to the west of the R.3. Hard*, ½ mile W of Castletown, which is sheltered by Chesil Beach and land from W and S winds, but even so can be very rough during gales. Yachtsmen are allowed to land on the RNSA (Portland Branch) pontoons close to the Castle. That is best bet of all, being adjacent to pubs and shops, so it is worth asking for a temporary berth. Castletown pier is private, and there is no public landing except on the beach just E of it. To the N and W of the pier there is a helicopter landing approach area: note the Prohibited Area shown on the harbour plan. If in doubt

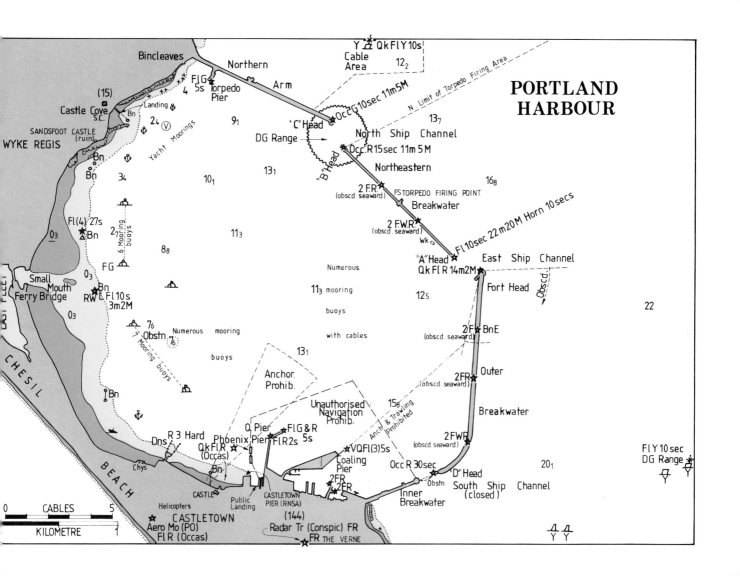

PORTLAND HARBOUR

Bincleaves

Northern Arm

Y QkFlY 10s
Cable Area   12₂

N. Limit of Torpedo Firing Area

Fl G
4 5s Torpedo Pier

Landing

(15)

Castle Cove S.C.

Bn

SANDSFOOT CASTLE (ruin)

WYKE REGIS

2₄ Ⓥ

Yacht Moorings

9₁

"C" Head

DG Range

OccG10sec 11m5M

13₇

North Ship Channel

"B" Head

Occ.R15sec 11m 5M

Northeastern

Bn

Bn

3₄

10₁

13₁

16₈

Fl(4)27s
Bn

11₃

2 F.R.
(obscd. seaward)

F S TORPEDO FIRING POINT

Breakwater

6 mooring buoys

8₈

2₇

FG

2 F.W.R.
(obscd. seaward)

Wk

Fl 10sec 22m20M Horn 10 secs

Small Mouth
Ferry Bridge

Bn

RW L Fl 10s
3m2M

0₃

0₃

Numerous

11₃ mooring

buoys

with cables

"A" Head
Qk Fl R 14m2M

East Ship Channel

Fort Head

Obscd

12₅

22

Obstn.

7₆

Numerous   mooring

buoys

2/F BnE
(obscd. seaward)

Bn

13₁

Anchor. Prohib.

Unauthorised Navigation Prohib.

15₈

Anch. & Trawling Prohibited

2FR
(obscd. seaward) Outer

Breakwater

2 FWR
(obscd. seaward)

Fl Y 10 sec
DG Range

R 3 Hard
Dns

QkFlR
(Occas)

Q Pier

Phoenix Pier

Fl G & R
5s

Fl R 2s

V QFl(3)5s

Coaling Pier

Occ R 30sec

D" Head

20₁

South Ship Channel
(closed)

Chys

Bn

CASTLE

2 FR
2 FR

Inner Breakwater

Obstn.

Public Landing

CASTLETOWN PIER (RNSA)

Helicopters

CASTLETOWN

(144)

Aero Mo (PO)
Fl R (Occas)

Radar Tr (Conspic) FR

FR THE VERNE

0   CABLES   5

KILOMETRE   1

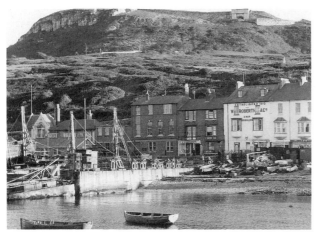

28.1 *Castletown Beach public landing-place*

contact the QHM at the Naval Base on Ch 13 or 14.

Facilities At Castletown. Water obtainable from Royal Breakwater Hotel or public houses. Fuel from garages at Victoria Sq., ¼ mile distant. PO and shops. EC Wed. Grocers, Sat. Banks and wider range of shops at Fortuneswell, ½ mile distant. Yacht yards at Ferrybridge. Launching site: rather restricted but light boats can be launched from Castletown beach, road adjacent, or from beach adjacent to bridge at Wyke Regis which joins mainland to Chesil causeway. Yacht clubs: Castle Cove SC, RNSA (Portland Branch).

Weather BBC Shipping forecast area: Portland.
Weymouth Bay Rdo Ch 05 at 0833, 2033.
Marinecall tel. 0898–500457.
BBC Rdo Devon 990 kHz (303m) at 0605, 0833, 1310, 1733 (not Sat). Sun 0833, 1310.

*29 Bridport

Charts: BA 3315; Im C5; Stan 12

High Water   −05h. 11m. Dover.
Heights above Datum   *In approach approx. MHWS 4m1. MLWS 0m6. MHWN 3m0. MLWN 1m6.*
Depths   *Bar within entrance between piers dries out. From 0m6 to 4m3 within harbour, but most parts dry out, except for the (3m3) coaster berths alongside and their turning area.*

WEST BAY, which is the port of Bridport, suffers from being a shallow artificial harbour which has a long narrow entrance. The entrance is dangerous in hard onshore weather. Once inside the harbour a yacht may be weather-bound waiting for fair conditions before attempting to leave, but this old West Country port is worth a visit, and offers a pleasant break on a passage across West Bay. There is some coastal trade.

Near LWS the inner sluice gates are opened and the entrance is scoured with the water released.

Approach and Entrance The approach to Bridport harbour is simple enough as far as outlying dangers are concerned, but the harbour entrance is unsafe in strong onshore winds, even at HW. Entry should be within 2 hours of HW.

When a vessel is expected and when there is sufficient depth a pilot flag is hoisted on the flagstaff above HM's office at the foot of the W pier; when the entrance is considered unsafe a B ball is hoisted. These signals are hoisted only for ships and not for yachts.

There is a Y can sewer buoy ½ mile SSW of the entrance to seaward of the 10m contour.

From S to E, steer straight for the entrance and, with sufficient tide, enter, but beware of the backwash off the piers.

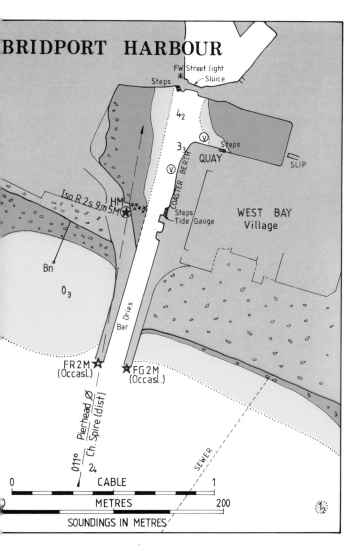

BRIDPORT HARBOUR

FW Street light
Sluice
Steps

4₂

Ⓥ Steps

3₃ QUAY

SLIP

Ⓥ COASTER BERTH

Iso R 2s 9m 5M

HM ✳✳✳

Steps
Tide Gauge

WEST BAY
Village

Bn

0₃

Dries

Bar

★ FR 2M
(Occasl.)

★ FG 2M
(Occasl.)

011° Pierhead ⌀
Ch. Spire (dist)

2₄

SEWER

0   CABLE   1
METRES   200
SOUNDINGS IN METRES

The recognized line of approach is W pierhead and the distant Bridport Church tower in line at 011°. The bar lies within the entrance and dries out but carries 3m or more at MHWS. The channel is long and narrow (14m) and boats without motors should be towed or rowed in. HW stands for 1½hrs.

Lights   The entrance should not be attempted by strangers at night. A Lt Iso R 9m 5M is established on HM's office at the root of the W pier. When a coaster is expected pilot Lts are exhibited: F G on E pierhead and F R on W pierhead, 3m 2M.

Day Signals   B ball – port closed
R flag with W cross – port open.

Anchorages and Moorings

(1) *Outside* the harbour in settled weather with offshore winds. Anchor about cable off the entrance in 2m4 clear of leading lines and sewer or to seaward in deeper water.

(2) *Inside the harbour* consult the HM on Ch 16, 11, 12 or 14. Small yachts dry out at the W end of the harbour, or alongside the harbour walls. There are coaster berths (3m3) alongside northern end of the E quay where scour from sluice makes a deep hole. Apply to the HM for the use of one, which he permits when no coaster is expected. Otherwise berth at E end of harbour drying alongside quay, soft mud bottom. HM tel. 0308–23222 – by night on 24977.

Facilities   Water from hydrants near the quay. Diesel and petrol at local garage. Shops, hotels and stores. EC Thurs. Scrubbing inside harbour; no yacht yard. Launching site: good slip and adjacent car park. Good bus connections to Bridport (1½ miles).

Weather   BBC forecast area: Portland.
Marinecall tel. 0898–500 457/458.
BBC Rdo Devon: 990kHz 0605, 0633, 0833, 1310, 1733.
Devonair Rdo: 666kHz 0715, 0745, 0845, 1730.
Start Point: VHF Ch 26 0803, 2003.

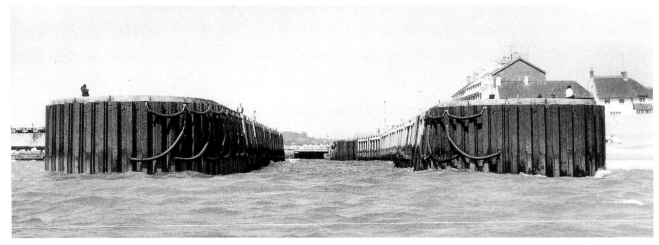

29.1 *Entrance near high water*

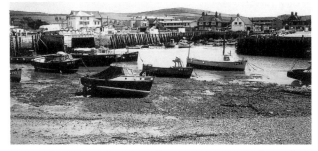

29.2 *The harbour dries out at low water except in the pool between the sluice on the left and the coaster berth to the right*

*30 Lyme Regis

Charts: BA 3315; Im C5; Stan 12

High Water —04h. 53m. Dover.
Heights above Datum *in approach approx. MHWS 4m3.
MLWS 0m6. MHWN 3m1. MLWN 1m7.*
   Depths *about 1m0 a cable east of the entrance at MLWS.
Harbour dries out at LW and entrance is less than 1m0, but there
is 4m0 at MHWS.*

LYME REGIS and its harbour, known as 'The Cobb', are
picturesque and worth visiting, though crowded in the holiday
season. The harbour dries out, but a berth alongside the quay is
sheltered from all but gales between NE and SE. In strong
onshore winds the approach and entrance are dangerous when
the swell enters the harbour.

Approach and Entrance Lyme Regis is just E of the
centre of Lyme Bay, some 22 miles W of Portland Bill. The
approach is straightforward. The harbour lies immediately S of
a conspicuous green parkland, marking the scene of a recent
landslip. It is protected from the W by the long stone pier known
as The Cobb, which is forked at its eastern end. To seaward of
the outer fork is a post and R can topmark marking a heap of
large Portland stones, serving as a breakwater and covered at
half flood. There are also stones and rocks all along the W and S
of The Cobb.

The entrance to the harbour lies between the eastern end of
the inner fork of The Cobb and the southern end of the detached
breakwater which affords partial protection to the harbour from
the E. The entrance is narrow.

Steer for the post and topmark off the outer fork of The Cobb,
leaving it about 50m to port and hold on until the harbour

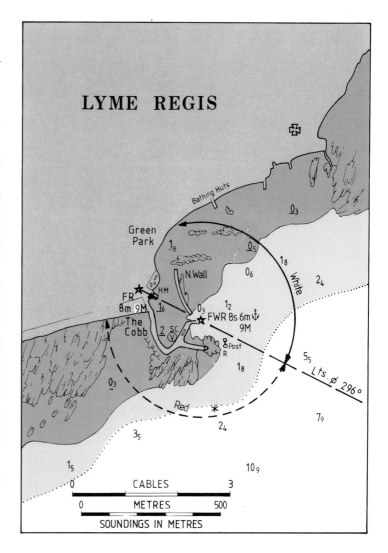

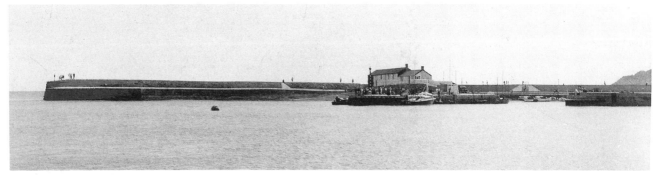

30.1 *Entrance from the eastward*

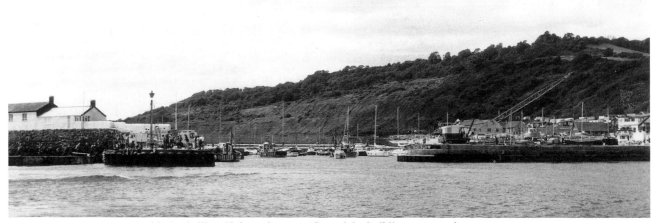

30.2 *Close to the entrance, with the Sailing Club on the upper floor of the building nearest the entrance*

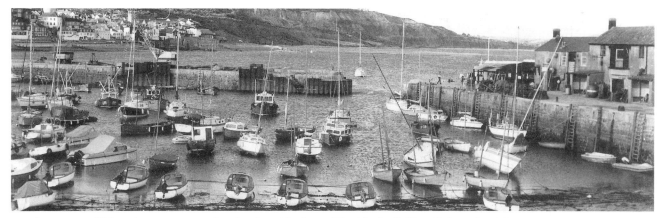

30.3 *Low water. Visitors have temporary berths alongside the wall beside the Sailing Club on the right*

entrance is opened up. Then steer in, given sufficient tide to enter the harbour. Usually all right ±3 hrs on HW.

Leading Lights   Front Lt on inner pierhead Oc W R 6m 9M. Rear light on old lamp-post above the HM's office and slipway F G 8m 9M. Lts in line lead in at 296°. The Lts are weak and often rendered inconspicuous by town lights.

Anchorages and Moorings

(1) Anchor *Outside the harbour* in settled weather and offshore winds to the E of the entrance. The anchor symbol on the plan shows the most northerly position in about 1m5 LAT, as the water shoals rapidly towards the shore. It is better to anchor in deeper water farther to seaward if remaining for any length of time, especially at Spring tides, but with less protection from the W. Take soundings to find the right depth; but it is better to consult the HM as the quality of the bottom varies.

(2) Most of the harbour dries out and the moorings in the centre are for permanent occupants. *At the quay alongside the sailing clubhouse* there are mooring berths for twelve visiting yachts only, but it is advisable to contact the HM in advance to reserve a berth on VHF Ch 16, 14 or telephone 029–742137. The innermost berth dries about 1m3 at LAT on clean sand bottom and the outer 0m3.

Facilities   Lyme Regis SC is on The Cobb on the floor above the aquarium. Bar open when G Lt is shown. Showers in boatshed. Water at shoreward end of The Cobb. Fuel delivered for a small fee. Hotels and shops. EC Thurs. Scrubbing can be arranged and small yacht repairs. Launching site, slip and car park adjacent. Dinghy park. Buses to all parts. Nearest station Axminster 6 miles.

Weather   See Bridport p. 173.
Shipping forecast area: Portland.

*31 Beer and Axmouth

IN NORTHERLY or north-westerly winds and settled weather there is a delightful anchorage for small yachts off BEER, 5 miles east of Sidmouth. It is sheltered by Beer Head, a precipitous headland (130m) easily identified as the most westerly white chalk cliff on the S Coast before the red cliffs of Devon. The anchorage is on the western side of the small bay east of the Head, as close inshore as soundings permit. Approaching from the W round Beer Head, follow the line of the cliffs, which have rocks at their base, until abreast of the road running down to the beach from the village with its conspicuous church with F W Lt near by (inconspic). Approaching from the E give a wide berth to the headland on the E side of the cove, which has rocks extending over a cable off it, before turning into the anchorage. Land by dinghy on beach, which is steep. Local fishermen and boatmen will ferry ashore.

With any forecast of change in wind leave quickly. Local fishing boats are hauled up on the beach out of danger. For yachts the nearest all-weather refuge is Brixham or Torquay.

Facilities Hotels, shops. EC Thurs. Boat-builder. Launching site from the road leading down to the beach.

Across Seaton Bay 1½ miles to the E of Beer Roads, the RIVER AXE runs into the sea close west of Haven Cliff. The entrance runs NNE, but is extremely narrow and marked only by a Fl 5s. light at its entrance, so it should be attempted only in calm weather and with local knowledge, preferably in a dinghy for the first time. Once inside, the river affords good shelter for boats drawing less than 1m5 which can take the ground at LW. Across the river ¼ mile from the entrance there is a low bridge, which impedes further navigation.

Facilities Axe YC, launching slip, boatyard, shops, hotels and PO. Occasional buses.

*32 Exmouth and River Exe

Charts: BA 2290; Im Y43, 65; Stan 12

High Water *Exmouth Dock.* −04h. 53m. *Dover. At Topsham* ½h. *later.*

Heights above Datum *Approaches MHWS 4m0. MLWS 0m2. MHWN 2m8. MLWN 1m3. Dock about 0m5 less.*

Depths *The approach and sands are liable to change, and the buoys are moved to conform. The depth of the bar is about 1m5 (2m0 MLWS). Within the harbour the bottom is uneven. There are deep stretches off Exmouth town and S and SW of Bull Hill Bank, but on the W and N of the bank there are 1m5 patches. The channel shoals to 1m0 up to Topsham and dries out completely just short of the M5 bridge, beyond which several weirs prevent further passage. The Exeter Canal has a least depth of 18ft.*

THE RIVER EXE has well-marked navigable channels going six miles inland towards Exeter from Exmouth. It is well worth a diversion during a West Country cruise. The only harbour is the small tidal dock at Exmouth; it is fully utilized by coastal freighters and is not available to yachts, but there are several safe spots to anchor or pick up moorings. It should not be regarded as a port of refuge, as the sands on the bar are liable to shift, and there is a dangerous sea during strong onshore winds, especially on the ebb. Under average conditions the approach and entrance are relatively straightforward, being well buoyed. In a shoal-draft boat or at the right tides Topsham, where they once built ships which fought the Armada, merits a visit, if only to see the avocets and other wildfowl.

Approach and Entrance The outer Fairway buoy (Sph bell buoy RW Vert bands) is situated ½ mile SSW of Straight

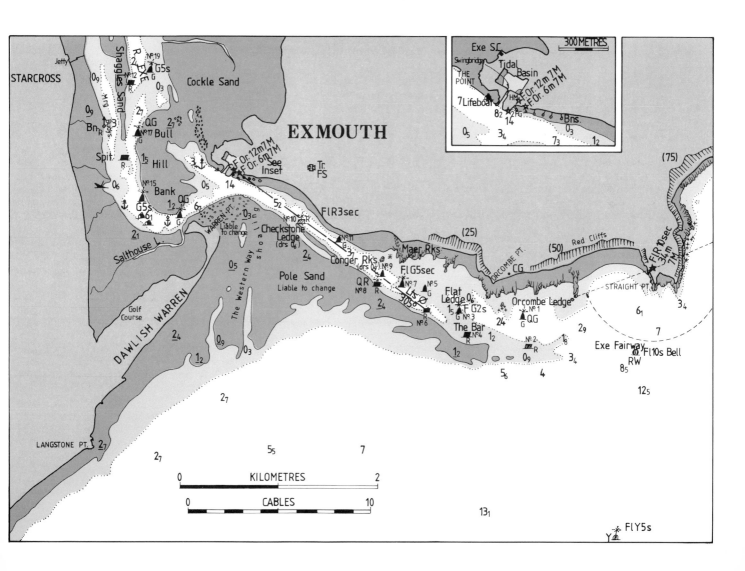

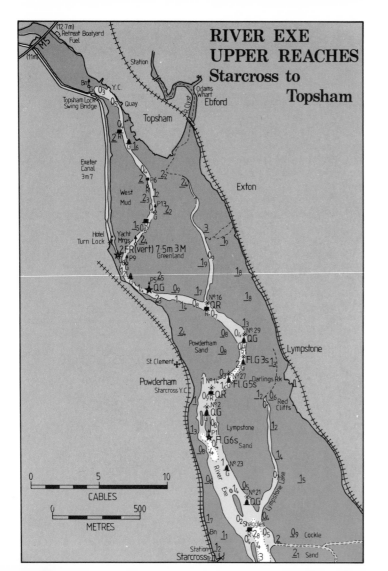

RIVER EXE
UPPER REACHES
Starcross to
Topsham

Point, which is a low promontory backed by R cliffs, but should not be confused with the lower Orcombe Point a mile westward. There are high cliffs between the two with ledges of rock at their foot. Whatever the direction of the approach, make for the Fairway buoy, but when coming from the direction of Torbay or Teignmouth give a good offing to the Pole sands, on the S side of the entrance channel, which are extending eastwards.

The entrance should not be attempted during strong onshore winds especially on the ebb. The best time to approach is half flood. This coincides with the turn of the offshore stream to the W. The tidal streams in the offing are weak but very strong in the channel and the entrance. As the sands are liable to shift after gales it is necessary to navigate up the channel by the buoys (which are moved accordingly), leaving the even-numbered R can buoys to port and the odd-numbered G con buoys to starboard. The leading marks on course 305° are difficult to pick up by day (FS on Customs House at rear and B post on the seawall at the front) or by night, when they tend to be lost in the town's lights. Some of the porthand buoys are very close to the Pole sands so they should not be approached too closely. The stream runs fiercely after the last port buoy (No. 10) has been

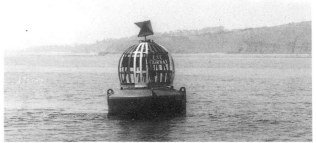

32.1 *Exmouth fairway bell buoy (safe water marking)*

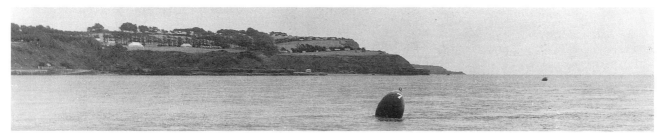

32.2 *View to seaward from No. 7 buoy, with Straight Point beyond*

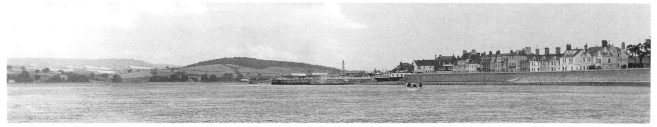

32.3 *Passing Checkstone Ledge buoy (No. 10) with Exmouth seafront on right*

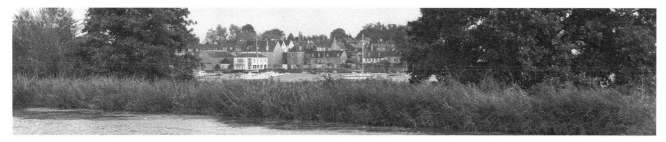

32.4 *A glimpse of Topsham from the Exeter Canal*

passed and it is best to keep on the starboard side of the fairway.

The River Off Exmouth the river takes a sharp turn to the SW (between Bull Hill Bank in the middle of the harbour and the Warren sands (the low point on the S side of the entrance). The main flood sweeps past Exmouth in a north-westerly direction and accordingly course should be altered sharply to port well before reaching the dock in order to get into the stream between Bull Hill Bank and the Warren Sands, and in particular to avoid the shoals extending E from Bull Hill Bank. The reach of the river S of the Bull Hill Bank is called the Bight and is marked by two starboard-hand buoys and by mooring buoys on the port hand. The channel follows round Bull Hill Bank northward and bends, leaving the R spit buoy and the Shaggles Sand to port and No. 17 buoy close to starboard. Unless heading for an anchorage off Starcross pier, follow Imray chart Y43 or BA 2290 heading towards Lympstone church tower 1½ miles to the NNE, passing between No. 12 R portland and No. 19 G starboard buoys. The channel then bears in a NNW direction towards Powderham, leaving to starboard No. 21, No. 23 G buoys and perch, soon bearing NNE again leaving to port Powderham Pool and No. 14 R buoy. Then follow the buoys in a shoaling channel with depths as low as 1m5 in parts nearly to Turf Lock. Above Turf Lock the channel is marked by Bns or buoys on either side as far as Topsham.

When proceeding from Exmouth up the river a considerable saving can be made by passing through the Shelly Gut. This is a shallow channel on the E side of Bull Hill Bank but it can be used only with local knowledge, as the sands are steep-to on either side and the channel is intricate.

The Starcross channel lies W of the Shaggles Sand and carries 0m9 to 2m1 as far as Starcross. It is entered at the Shaggles Spit R buoy (leaving it to starboard). Although the channel is unmarked except by a Bn on the port side, the best water can be located by the larger yachts lying on moorings in it.

Lights Straight Point Lt Fl R 10s. 34m 9M. Exe Fairway buoy Fl 10s. (bell).

The approach is marked by Fl or Q G Lts on the starboard hand (which is the easier side to follow) and by Lts on two buoys (Q R and Fl R 3s.) on the port hand. There are two Lts, F Or 7M, near the Customs House and the dock which lead in line at 305°; but the transit crosses the outer end of the Pole Sands and is only of service from No. 6 porthand buoy (no light) to the Checkstone No. 10 porthand buoy Fl R 3s. For the first 2 miles (as far as Powderham) only starboard-hand channel buoys carry lights.

Anchorage and Moorings

(1) *Outside*, off the entrance, W of the Fairway buoy in calm weather.

(2) *Exmouth dock*. This is approached through a narrow entrance where ferries berth, and is spanned by a swingbridge which has to be opened by arrangement with the HM – on Ch 16 or 12 during office hours or by telephone 0395–272009. The basin is tidal. In 1990 it was reserved for commercial traffic.

(3) Anchor (if room can be found clear of moorings) *beyond the entrance to the dock off the Point* in 3m, clear of the lifeboat. Five-knot tidal stream at Spring tides; rough when wind against tide.

(4) Large yachts may anchor clear of the fairway in the *Bight between Bull Hill Bank and Warren Sands*.

(5) *West of Bull Hill Bank* outside the small craft moorings.

(6) Anchorage off *Starcross*, SE of the pier in 0m6 to 2m1 but best positions occupied by private moorings. Enquire at club for possible temporary vacancy. Well sheltered from W. Water, and some facilities. EC Thurs. Ferry to Exmouth. Main line station.

(7) There is a mooring area between the perch, No. 25 buoy and *Lympstone Sand* which is approached from No. 23 buoy and stated to have an approximate depth of 1m0 at LW.

(8) Small craft can anchor in 1m5 S of landing stage at *Turf Lock*

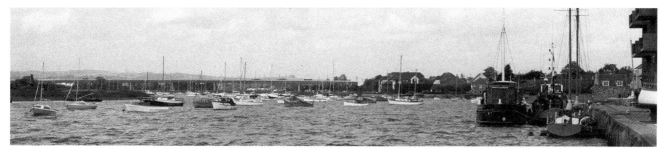

32.5 *Boats lying alongside The Quay at Topsham, M5 viaduct in the background*

clear of the coasters' fairway, or N of No. 25 buoy.

(9) At *Topsham* it is possible to anchor on the edge of the fairway which is immediately to the E of the line of moorings between the R pole P6 and a R can beyond the Quay. Or secure alongside the Quay (prominent redbrick warehouse) and take the bottom (soft mud) at LW. This has the advantage of being next to The Lighter Hotel which offers warm hospitality and imaginative food.

Access to Exeter by the Exeter Canal The Canal is 5 miles (8km) long. From the south it is entered at Turf Lock, where there is a good pub. Least depth 3m7. At the Exeter end there is a locked basin. Prior permission from the City Council (tel. 0392–74306) or by speaking to the lock-keeper. Headroom limit of 11m under the M5 1½ miles N of Turf, but small craft can go on to the pub at Double Lock or all the way to the Maritime Museum. Opposite Topsham there is an old lock-gate giving access to the Canal. It is due to be restored. When it is in use it will be possible to go up to Topsham about 2 hours before HW and later return along the Canal, waiting at Turf Lock if necessary for the tide. It is easier to park at Topsham and take the bus to Exeter.

Facilities at Exmouth and Topsham. Boat-builders and repairers. Customs. Water by hose at dock. Petrol and oil. Hotels and shops. EC Wed. Showers at yacht clubs.

Launching sites:
(1) Ramp S of harbour entrance near HW, where yacht club puts a wooden ramp over the soft sand in summer months; little room in road for cars and trailers but car park on the pier.
(2) Beach N of harbour entrance.
(3) By arrangement with yacht yards.
(4) At Lympstone, 2 miles N of Exmouth ramp, for launching near HW. Yacht clubs: Exe SC, Starcross YC at Powderham Pt, Starcross Fishing and Cruising Club at Starcross, Topsham SC, Lympstone SC.

Fuel There is only one alongside source of diesel on the River, which is at the pontoon of the Retreat Boatyard close to the M5. It is only accessible near HW. Otherwise fuel has to be humped on board in jerricans.

Railway and bus services on both sides of the River. Exeter Airport is near by. Further information about River, call Topsham 0392–873044.

Weather Forecast area Portland. See Bridport p. 173.

*33 Teignmouth

Charts: BA 26; Im Y43, C5; Stan 12

High Water *approaches* −05h. 11m. *Dover.*
Heights above Datum *MHWS 4m8. MLWS 0m6. MHWN 3m6. MLWN 1m9.*
Depths *About 0m3 on the bar; deep pool off Ferry Point, then depths in the fairway over 2m up to Shaldon bridge.*

TEIGNMOUTH is an attractive little seaside town. The harbour on the W and SW side is well sheltered, but the streams are fast so that it is best to obtain moorings if possible. The entrance is difficult for strangers and the bar makes it dangerous during onshore winds when a swell is running.

Approach and Entrance The entrance lies to the northward of the Ness, a bold R sandstone headland with pines at its summit, which is easy to identify. The Ness and the Pole Sands projecting eastward from it flank the S side of the river entrance, and the Spratt Sands lie on the N side. The sands on the bar are constantly shifting and in some years steep sandbanks build up.

Without a pilot or assistance from those with local knowledge the entrance should not be attempted by strangers, except with the utmost caution in settled weather during offshore winds and on the last quarter of the flood.

Approach from the southward with the *inner* end of the pier bearing about N magnetic. Before the Ness comes abeam identify the leading marks above the Point (grey stone tower at front, B pillar at rear) on a transit of 334°. This will lead over Pole Sands at a point which dries 0m3, thence into deeper water W of the bar and S of Spratt Sands.

To the W will now be seen the W Bn with a B base (Philip Lucette) on the NW side of the Ness, on a training wall which is covered before half flood. When this Bn bears between 250° and 258° steer about 40m off it, taking soundings to skirt the N side of the Pole Sands. An alternative and more direct approach is from the E steering on a steady bearing of 254° for the conspic WB Bn, leaving to port a Y con buoy about 1 cable NNE of The Ness, until altering to starboard off the Philip Lucette Bn and proceeding to round up towards Teignmouth as described below. Neither approach should be attempted at night or in fresh onshore winds. You may be lucky enough to coincide with the passage of a pilot-boat, but always remember that you will

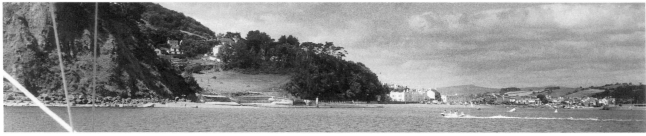

33.1 *Close to the Bar on a WSW'ly course. Philip Lucette beacon in centre. Shaldon on the right. The cliff on the left is The Ness*

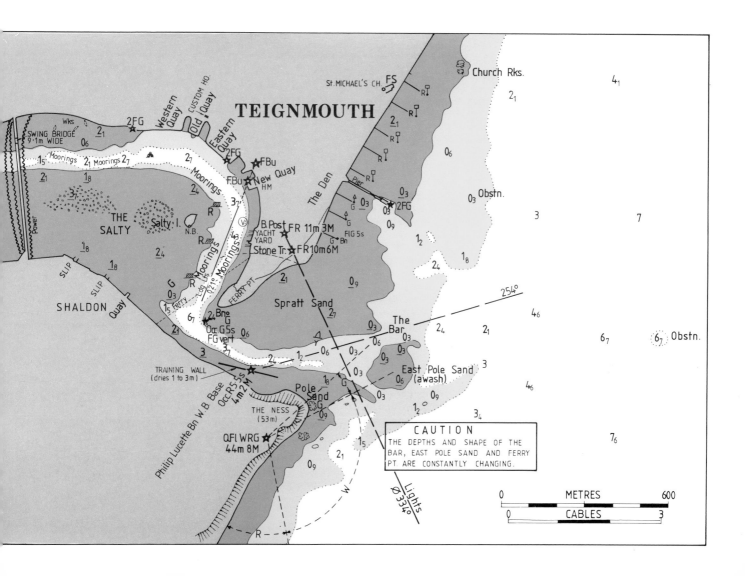

have to cross a patch which dires om3 at MLWS, so a stranger may have trouble finding the best water and the sands are liable to change. Leaving the WB Bn to port, come slowly to starboard so as to round the G Bn off Ferry Point on the N side of the channel. Note that the sands have extended from the point, so the Bn should left clear to starboard. Here the stream runs very hard. Once past Ferry Point alter course quickly to starboard to 021° and head for the end of the New Quay, leaving the three R can buoys well to port.

The whole of the centre of the harbour is occupied by 'The Salty' flat; the river runs round to its E. Pilotage is now easier because the flats are marked by porthand buoys, while the starboard shore is fairly steep-to. After passing the third R porthand buoy keep on the starboard side of the channel parallel to Eastern Quay until rounding into the straight E–W reach leading to the bridge. Here the direction of the channel can be judged by yachts lying on moorings, keeping close to the larger ones for the best water.

Lights   There is a sector Lt (Q WRG) on the Ness. Near the waterfront of the town there are F R leading Lts on 334° over the eastern extremity of Pole Sands, but strangers should not attempt the entrance at night; the leading lights are intended for those with local knowledge. Note that the Philip Lucette Bn is now all-round and not a sector Lt.

Anchorage and Mooring   Anchoring is possible outside Teignmouth harbour 1 to 2 cables SE of the pier end or a cable SE of the Ness in settled weather and offshore winds. Within the harbour it is difficult to anchor as the streams are strong and there are moorings and chains on the bottom in all the best parts. The only possibility is at Neap tides on the edge of The Salty near the second and third R buoys. Accordingly it is necessary to try to find a vacant mooring. There is a visitors' mooring off the yacht yard on the E side of the channel in deep water. Moor fore and aft to two R buoys with a 15m spread. Enquire of the HM at

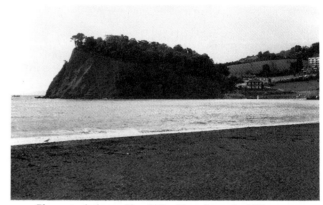

33.2 *Characteristic profile of The Ness from the NE*

New Quay for moorings temporarily vacant. Call on Ch 16 or 12 during office hours, or by telephone on 0626–773165.

Upper Reaches   The river above Shaldon Bridge is navigable as far as Newton Abbot at high water by small craft with local knowledge. Depth at bridge 2m0 at MHWS.

Facilities   Customs at Old Quay. Water from New Quay. Fuel and chandlery also available at Shaldon. Yacht yard with patent slipway up to 36m long and 2m7 draught, and two small boatyards. Several hotels and restaurants. Good shops. EC Thurs. Launching site for dinghies at Shaldon. At Teignmouth launching is possible at the end of Lifeboat Lane and Gales Hill, also at Pellew Steps, and there is a launching site at the yacht yard. Ferry to Shaldon. Yacht clubs: Teign Corinthian YC, Shaldon SC. Buses. Main line railway. NH racing at Newton Abbot 4 miles.

Weather   See Bridport p. 173.
Shipping forecast area: Portland.

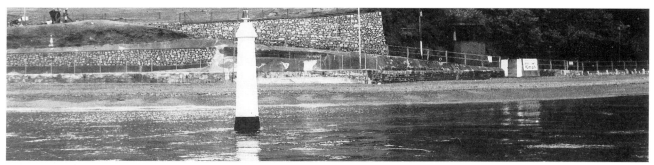

33.3 *Philip Lucette beacon, with 10-knot speed limit notice to the right. A white block of flats now dominates the background of this picture (see right of pic. 33.2)*

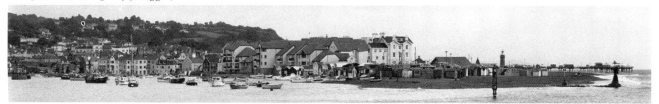

33.4 *Rounding up to moorings off Teignmouth. Note G beacon off Ferry Point and pleasure pier to seaward*

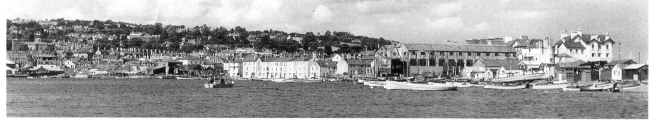

33.5 *On the NNE reach between The Salty and Teignmouth. Visitors' moorings off yacht yard on the right*

34 Torquay

Charts: BA 26; Im C5, Y43; Stan 12

High Water −05h. 08m. Dover.
Heights above Datum *MHWS 4m9. MLWS 0m7. MHWN 3m7. MLWN 2m0.*
Depths *4m2 just within the entrance. Inside the outer harbour there is over 3m alongside the Haldon (E) pier, and the Princess (W) pier. In the southern part of the harbour the depth is over 2m, but the inner harbour dries out except at the end of the S pier. Depths in the marina are from 2m0 to 1m5.*

TORQUAY lies in the north-western corner of Torbay, well sheltered, except from strong onshore winds. The town is a large and popular seaside resort and over-crowded during the holiday season. Its attraction for visiting yachtsmen has been greatly enhanced by the completion of a 500-berth marina with adequate car parking, all in a Côte d'Azur setting.

Approach and Entrance Approaching from the eastward, the church tower on high ground at the back of Babbacombe Bay and the spire of the Roman Catholic church will first be seen. Torbay will next be identified with Hope Nose and the Ore Stone (32m) and Thatcher (41m) rocks on the N side and Berry Head on the S. Entering the N side of the bay note that there is a rock awash about 90m SW of Ore Stone, and the Morris Rogue (0m8 over it) 1½ cables SE of the E Shag (11m) rock.

From the southward there are no outlying dangers. The entrance is 61m wide, and within the outer harbour there is plenty of water for yachts. There is not much room for manoeuvre, so enter slowly and be prepared to meet excursion vessels, which are frequently leaving the harbour. In an emergency there are traffic signals at the seaward end of Haldon Pier:

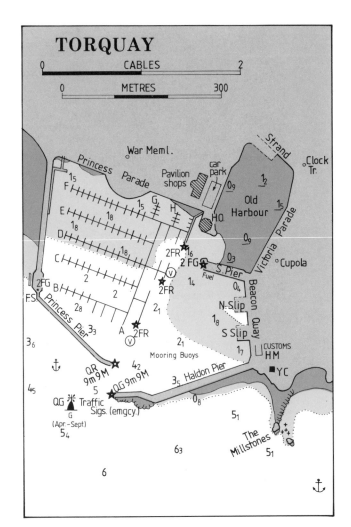

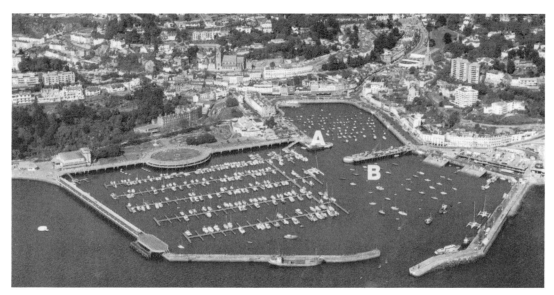

34.1 *(A) Harbour Office (B) Fuel dock*

3 R balls by day or 3 R Lts (Vert) by night.

Lights 90m W of the entrance a G con buoy Q G (April–Sept). On the Haldon (E) pierhead a Q G 9m 9M; and on the Princess (W) pierhead is a Q R 9m 9M. The outer end of the inner (S) pier is marked by two F G Vert. The three sets of 2F R Lts at the eastern end of each pontoon of the marina are the port-hand channel markers leading in to the Old Harbour.

Anchorage and berths

(1) *Outside the harbour* in offshore winds there is good holding ground off Princess pier in 3m6 minimum, or near the end of Haldon pier in 2m4, but keep clear of the fairway with its frequent ferry traffic.

(2) *Inside the harbour* make for one of the visitors' berths on the marina at its SE extremity and call the office on Ch 37. The HM on Ch 16 during office hours might direct you to one of his moorings or allow a temporary berth alongside Haldon pier.

Facilities The marina (tel. 0803–214624/5), which always keeps 60 visitors' berths available, has everything, including shore power, water and fuel, showers, launderette, repair facilities, bar-restaurant, car parking. By permission of the HM (tel. 0803–292429) use of the slips at the eastern end of the harbour can be obtained. Torquay has plenty of 4-star hotels at 5-star prices. Restaurants and shopping to cater for all. Buses. The main-line railway station has frequent intercity expresses. There is a ferry running across to Brixham and sightseeing trips up the Dart. The R. Torbay YC overlooks the end of Haldon pier.

Weather See Plymouth p. 220.
Shipping forecast area: Portland.
Marinecall tel. 0898–500. 458.
Start Point: VHF Ch 26 0803, 2003.
BBC Rdo Devon: 1458kHz 0605, 0833, 1310, 1733.
Devonair Rdo: 954kHz 0715, 0745, 0815, 0845, 1730.

*35 Paignton

PAIGNTON has a very small harbour on the W side of Torbay, N of Roundham Head, with its prominent red cliffs. From the E quay with its Lt Fl R 7m 3M there is a rocky outcrop running due E, the seaward extremity of which is marked by a R lattice Bn with a spoil ground topmark. Approach from NE is simplest.

The harbour dries out and is crowded with moorings but there is good anchorage in offshore winds north-east of the entrance within easy reach of the harbour by dinghy. Facilities are good and the HM can sometimes arrange a berth where a visiting yacht can dry out alongside the quay.

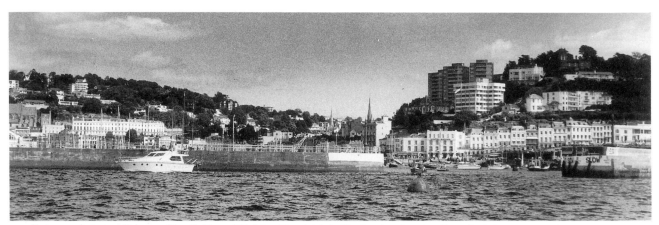

34.2 *Entrance between Princess Pier (left) and Haldon Pier (right). Marina berths are all on the left*

36 Brixham

Charts: BA 26; Im Y43, C5; Stan 12

High Water −0.5h. 11m. Dover.
Heights above Datum MHWS 4m7. MLWS 0m7. MHWN 3m4. MLWN 1m9.
Depths *The outer harbour is deep but the inner harbour dries out at Springs almost to the end of the New pier.*

BRIXHAM's history features two notable Royal arrivals by sea. In 1688 William of Orange became the last successful invader of England when he landed there to claim its crown. In 1815 the Emperor Napoleon Bonaparte was brought to Torbay in HMS *Bellerephon* as a prisoner awaiting a decision on his next move. From here hundreds of those fast and sea-kindly Brixham trawlers ranged far and wide to make offshore fishing a major industry. After Hitler's war the fleet never recovered until it enjoyed a sharp revival in the late 1960s. A new deep-draught fishing harbour was built outside the drying inner harbour. Now up to 50 large trawlers use Brixham Fish Harbour. This has also seen a mass return of fat incontinent seagulls from Berry Head who are no respecters of gleaming teak decks. In 1989 the 500-berth Prince William Marina was built in the SE corner of the outer harbour, with access to big yachts at all states of the tide. It is protected from the NE by a wave-screen wrapped around the pontoons.

The outer harbour is readily accessible at all states of the tide and has moorings either side of the fairway. The Brixham YC has its own pontoons off the steps leading up to the clubhouse and welcomes visitors.

Approach and Entrance Brixham lies a mile W of Berry Head, which is a prominent headland sloping at 45°. The

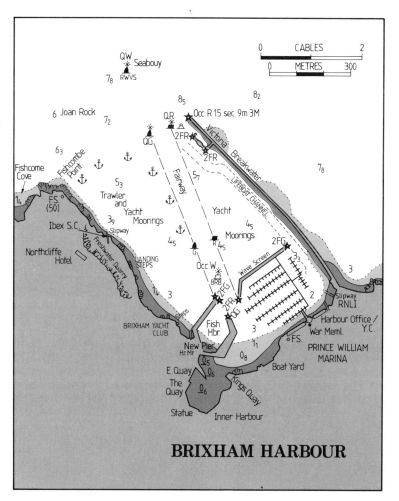

BRIXHAM HARBOUR

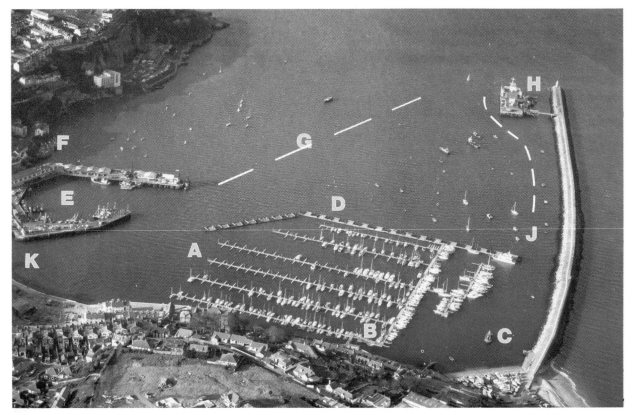

36.1 *Brixham Harbour facing NW. (A) Prince William Marina (B) Marina Office (C) Lifeboat (D) Wave-screen (E) Commercial Fishing Harbour (F) Brixham YC (G) Main fairway (155°) (H) Commercial oil jetty at seaward end of Victoria Bkwtr (J) Lifeboat channel (K) Entrance to Inner Harbour*

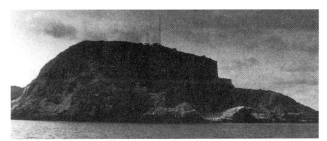

36.2 *Berry Head with coastguard and radio mast above old quarries, heading WNW towards harbour entrance on the right*

harbour entrance is wide, but it should not be cut close to on entering, due to the constant traffic of tripper and fishing boats. There is a RWVS safe water buoy (Q W) a cable off the end of the breakwater which should be left to the south. Speed limit is 5 kts. The only snag is that access by road is difficult, especially during the summer.

Lights Berry Head Lt, Gp Fl (2) 15s. 58m 18M. At end of breakwater Lt Oc R 15s. 6M. Seabuoy Q W.

Anchorages

(1) *Outside in Brixham Roads* in about 7m, or small yachts can anchor in fine weather outside to the E of the breakwater, close in towards Shoalstone Point.

(2) *Inside on W side of the harbour* as indicated on the plan, between moorings and just clear of fairway. Inevitably there is often considerable wash from passing trawlers and excursion boats near the fairway, so it is preferable to be close to the land near the entrance in reasonable weather.

(3) Small yachts can anchor in *Fishcombe Cove* (just W of the headland at entrance) but this position can be dangerous if the wind freshens anywhere N to NE.

(4) In the E side of the harbour to the NW of the Marina wavescreen.

(5) Prince William Marina has 535 berths including visitors' for boats up to 35m LOA and drawing 3m. Contact on Ch 16, 37 or 80, tel. 0803–882711.

(6) Berths for commercial FV have been provided at new basin in SW corner near the Fishmarket.

There are some visitors' mooring buoys in the harbour, but if none is found vacant apply to HM or the boatman at the yacht club. Yachts should be reported to the HM within 24 hours of arrival. In the event of gales from the NW or N, shelter should be sought elsewhere. The Marina is fully protected.

The HM is on Ch 14 or 16; tel. 08045–3321. Berthing master: 08045–3211.

Facilities Brixham is well provided with facilities for visiting yachts. There are banks, hotels, restaurants and shops of all kinds (EC Wed.). There is a boatyard with four slipways and 10-ton hoist. Two other boat repairers. Two scrubbing grids 2m4 draught and eight scrubbing berths 3m0 draught by arrangement with HM. Also crane lift 4 tons at quay head. Compass swinging by arrangement with HM. Sailmakers. Water is obtainable by permission at the yacht club steps or at the New pier where diesel oil is also obtainable. Customs Office. Yacht chandlers at quay and at Marina, where there are full facilities, including showers, clubhouse. There are also luxury apartments overlooking the Marina. Launching sites: from SE corner of outer harbour at all states of tide, breakwater hard slipway and from new slipway at Freshwater Quarry. Frequent buses to all parts and excursion boats to Torquay and Paignton. Yacht clubs: Brixham YC, Ibex SC, Castle Rock YC, at Marina.

Coastguards on Berry Head are on VHF Ch 16, 10; 67. Tel. 08045–58292.

Weather See Torquay p. 190.

Shipping forecast area: Portland (Plymouth).

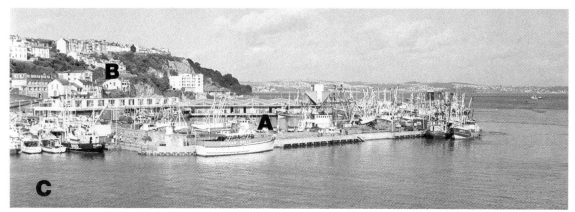

36.3 *(A) Busy new fishing harbour as seen from Marina (B) Brixham YC (C) Entrance to Old Harbour*

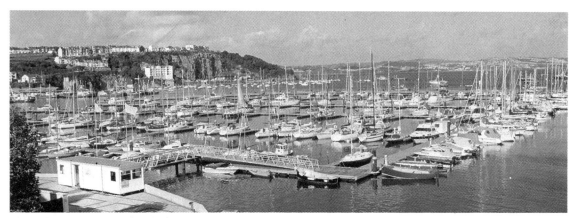

36.4 *Prince William Marina facing north-west, with boats on swinging moorings beyond*

37 Dartmouth

Charts: BA 2253; Im Y47; Stan 12

High Water   −05h. 15m. Dover.
Heights above Datum   MHWS 4m8. MLWS 0m4. MHWN
3m6. MLWN 1m8.
Depths   *Deep water channel as far as Dittisham; beyond there are considerable variations in depth.*

DARTMOUTH is best known today as the home of the Royal Naval College, but the town's unspoilt 16th-century buildings evoke a maritime past when it rated above Plymouth in importance. It is one of the best-protected harbours on the S Coast, perfectly set on steep-to cliffs running down each side to the Dart, which is navigable as far as Totnes, 10 miles inland. Returning from a cruise to Brittany, W Cork or Spain, one wonders why one ever sailed away, for there is no more beautiful harbour. It always has room for visiting yachts of any size or draught.

Approach and Entrance   Dartmouth lies 5 miles W of Berry Head and 7 miles N of Start Point (see pages 35 and 36, in Passage Data section). The entrance is not conspicuous from seaward, but it can be located by the conspicuous 24m daymark (elevation 170m) above Froward Point, E of the entrance, and the craggy Mewstone Rock (35m).

The entrance is deep and well marked but there are dangers. On the E side there are rocks to the W of the Mewstone; the Verticals (dry 1m8) and the W Rock with a depth over it of 0m9. Off Inner Froward Pt is the Bear's Tail (dries 0m6) and 2¼ cables W is Old Castle Rock (with 1m8 over it), marked by the G con Castle Ledge buoy (Fl G 5s.). From about 3 hours flood to 3 hours ebb the stream sets towards these dangers, which should

be given a wide berth. Approaching from the eastward keep the East Blackstone Rock (which is ½ mile E of Mewstone) well open of the Mewstone until the G con Castle Ledge buoy comes in line with Blackstone Pt on the W side of the entrance.

On the W side there are rocks a cable off Combe Point; 3 cables off this Pt is the Homestone (with 0m9), marked by R can buoy. Further towards the mouth of the river are the Meg Rocks which dry 3m0 and the Western Blackstone Rock (2m high).

Between these dangers the fairway is wide and the approach is easy, except in strong S or SE winds when a heavy swell runs into the harbour, at times as far as the lower ferry. Meeting an *ebb* tide it can cause an ugly sea for small vessels. In the narrows there are two rocks to avoid on the W side opposite Kingswear Castle, the Checkstone (0m3 over it) and the Kitten rock (1m8) SSE of the R can Checkstone buoy (Fl (2) R 5s.) which lies off the ledges on the western side. The Kitten rock is on the edge of the fairway, so when approaching the narrows keep E of it and give a good berth to the Checkstone buoy.

At night keep in the W sector of the Iso WRG 3s. 9m 8M light on the Kingswear side in a squat W tower. Past the two castles and a cable beyond the Checkstone buoy come round to 293° in the middle of the river in the W sector of the Bayards Cove Lt (Fl WRG 2s. 5m 6M) identifiable by day by a W stripe on the rock of the foreshore on the Dartmouth side. Proceed upharbour in mid-stream. When outward bound, there is a F W 5m 9M light just up-river of Kingswear Castle visible 102°–107°.

Anchorage and Moorings

(1) *Outside* there is a temporary anchorage in settled weather in the range but there is often an uncomfortable swell. It is prohibited in the area between Blackstone Pt bearing 291° and Combe Pt bearing 343° owing to cables which emerge seaward from Compass Cove.

(2) Anchorage available east of *main channel opposite Dartmouth* between line of large buoys and small craft moorings, but

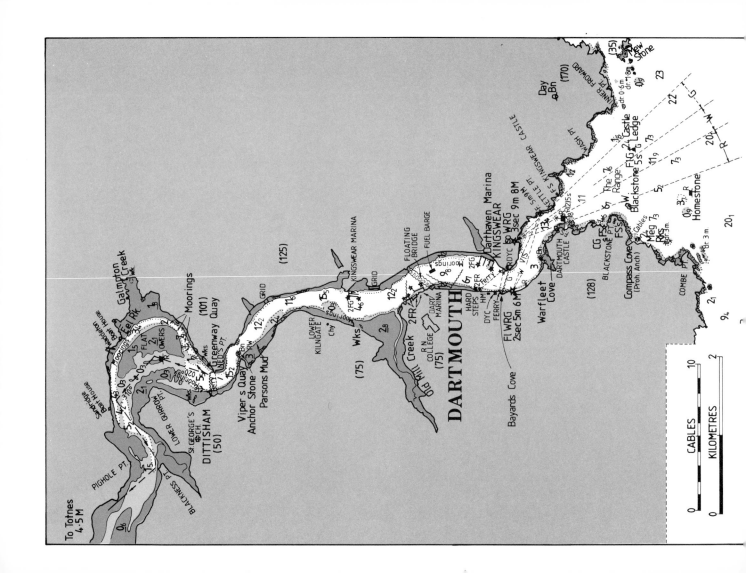

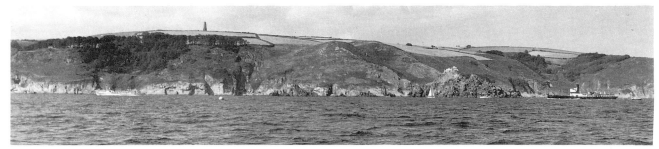

37.1 *Dartmouth day beacon bearing north seen from one mile offshore*

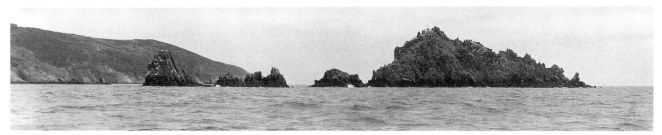

37.2 *Mewstone from the south-west*

beware of ground chain. The Royal Dart YC has six moorings, which may be used by visitors on application to the Club.

(3) *Dart Harbour and Navigation Commission moorings* are marked DHC and are on the E side of the harbour with some for smaller yachts on the Dartmouth side, on application to the HM on Ch 11 or tel. 08043–2337. Berthing for short periods is allowed alongside the embankment wall, where there is also a scrubbing grid.

(4) Alongside at the *Darthaven Marina* just upstream of Kingswear Railway Station. Contact on Ch 37 or tel. 080425–545.

(5) Moorings and berths at *Dart Marina* above floating bridge on W side, with petrol, diesel oil, water, yacht yard, hotel and all facilities. Tel. 08043–3351. The same organization also has berths alongside the Kingswear Marina up-river off Noss Works. Contact both on Ch 37.

(6) There are temporary public pontoons near the lower car ferry and off Coombe Park just downstream of Dart Marina.

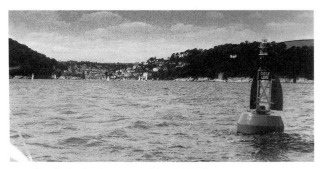

37.3 *Castle Ledge buoy, 6 cables SSE of entrance*

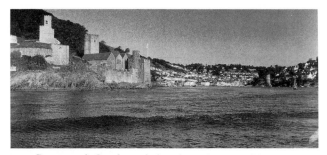

37.4 *Dartmouth Castle and church on the west side of the entrance*

(7) *Off Parsons Mud* on the W side of the river south of the Anchor Stone, but cargo ships proceed all the way up the river and the channel must be kept clear at all times.

(8) *Greenway Quay*, Dittisham. Some visitors' moorings off Ferry Boat Inn at Dittisham and off Stoke Gabriel. Anchor off Ferry Boat Inn below moorings. Fresh water tap on quay in front of inn. LW landing pontoon at Dittisham for dinghies. Small passenger ferry operates between Dittisham and Greenway. Scrubbing alongside Greenway Quay by arrangement with ferry operator. Yacht yards in Galmpton Creek. Also anchorages off the upper boathouse between Sandridge Pt and Galmpton Creek and upstream beyond Blackness Pt.

Upper Reaches   (a) If proceeding up river from Dittisham to the east of Flat Owers Bank, keep all mooring buoys close to starboard to avoid the mudbank. (b) When there is sufficient water to navigate to the W of the Flat Owers Bank, steer for the boathouse at Waddeton until the R buoy is abeam to port, then alter course to port and steer for the upper Sandridge boathouse. When the upper Sandridge boathouse is abeam to starboard, alter for Blackness Pt, keeping Higher Gurrow Pt fairly close to

port. When Blackness Pt is abeam to port, alter for Pighole Pt and leave all moorings close to starboard after passing Pighole Pt. (c) If proceeding beyond Stoke Gabriel, when Mill Pt is abeam alter for the middle of the wood on the S bank of the river. Off the entrance to Bow Creek there are R and G channel buoys, then steer for the R buoy off Duncannon. The river is marked with buoys and Bns to the end of the Fleet Mill Reach after which the best water is in the centre of the river to Totnes.

Make fast alongside in the Mill Tail which is the left-hand channel on arrival at Totnes. The main river has two trots of moorings and a visitors' mooring is sometimes available by arrangement with the Totnes Boating Association. The Mill Tail dries out, the bottom being mud to a depth of about 0m5 and then sand. Attractive old town with castle. Boatyard. Chandlery. Hotels and restaurants. Shops.

Facilities   Water by arrangement at Harbour Office or at any marina. At Dittisham public standpipes. Fuel at marinas and from a barge moored in the middle of the river between the upper and lower ferries (Contact on Ch 16). Hotels and restaurants, good shopping centre – EC part Wed. part Sat.

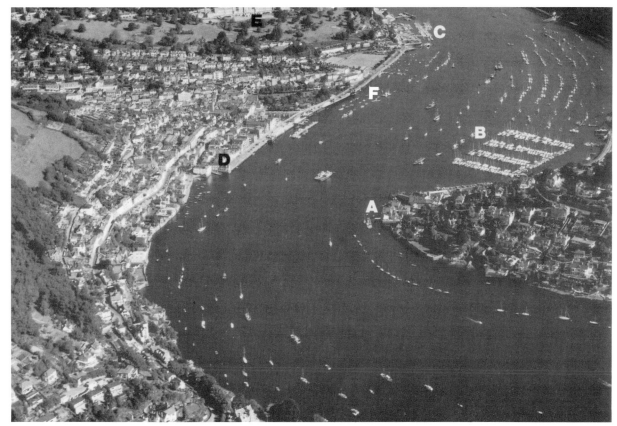

37·5 *(A) Royal Dart Yacht Club (B) Darthaven Marina (C) Dart Marina (D) Harbour Office with temporary waiting pontoons (E) Royal Naval College (F) Public pontoons*

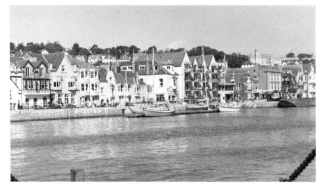

37.6 *Waiting pontoon near Dartmouth Harbour Office upstream from the Kingswear car ferry. Royal Naval College on skyline top right*

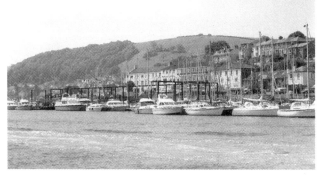

37.7 *Darthaven Marina alongside old Kingswear railway yard*

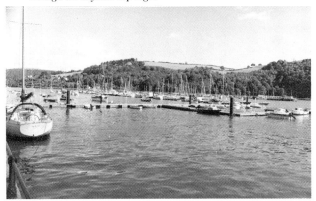

37.8 *Dartmouth public pontoons just downstream of floating-bridge chain ferry*

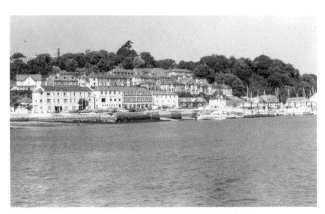

37.9 *Dart Marina with floating-bridge slip on left and RN College clocktower on skyline*

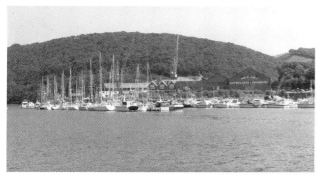

Customs House. Yacht yards, chandlers and all facilities. Travel-hoist at Darthaven Marina. Yacht clubs: R. Dart YC (Kingswear), Dartmouth YC, Dittisham SC. Launching sites: public slipway at Kingswear next R. Dart YC, except near LW. Slipway at Dartmouth dinghy basin, 2 hours each side HW or at any tide from slipway alongside upper ferry slipway, provided ferry is not obstructed. The nearest rail connection is at Paignton 7 miles away. Buses to all parts.

Weather   See Torquay p. 190.

BBC shipping forecast area: Portland (Plymouth)

37.10 *Kingswear Marina upstream on site of Philip's yard*

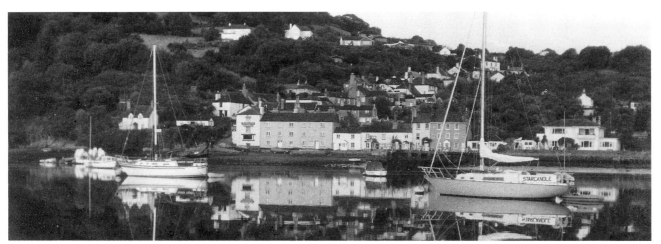

37.11 *Anchorage off Dittisham on the west bank, 3 miles upstream from the entrance to the River Dart. Ferry slip on the left*

*38 Salcombe

Charts: BA 28; Im Y48; Stan 13

High Water   −05h. 38m. Dover.
Heights above Datum   MHWS 5m3. MLWS 0m7. MHWN 4m1. MLWN 2m1.
Depths   *On the leading marks the bar normally has a depth of 1m5, but immediately E of the transit there is only 0m7 and the depth on the bar sometimes changes. Above the bar there is a deep channel as far as Tosnos Pt in the 'Bag'. From there to Heath Pt there is upwards of 2m with local knowledge, but strangers may not find more than 1m2 in parts. The estuary then shallows, but at three-quarters flood it is possible for vessels of 2m7 draught to navigate up to Kingsbridge, some 3 miles above Salcombe.*

VISITING yachtsmen consider this lovely well-sheltered estuary to be one of the best of the West Country ports. It offers safe anchorages and some visitors' moorings, and is ideal for day sailing, picnics and walks.

Approach and Entrance   The entrance is simple with sufficient tide on the bar and in settled weather. During strong onshore winds it can be dangerous.

It lies just to the E of Bolt Head, and some 3 miles W of the Prawle. Bolt Head is a remarkable promontory with a spiked skyline. There are two islets, the Mewstone (19) and Little Mewstone (5), off the Point.

Strong southerly winds meeting the ebb at the Bolt set up overfalls which can be avoided by approaching from farther E. The only dangers in the approach are rocks to the W near the Mewstones, and on the E side of the Rickham Rock, which has 2m7 over it. It is simplest to alter course northward about ¼ mile

E of the Bolt. Now sail past Starehole Bay where the remains of the wreck of the barque *Herzogin Cecilie* lie in the NW corner under the high cliffs.

A headland on the NE corner of this little bay with a detached rock (the Great Eelstone) and Cadmus Rocks (0m3) S of it must be avoided. The bar is 2 cables N of the Great Eelstone Rock which must be left about 1½ cables to port. The leading marks on 360° consist of a RW Bn with RW cage topmark on the Poundstone Rock (dries 4m) and a RW Bn with a diamond topmark on Sandhill Pt (Dir Fl WRG 2s. 27m 10M) situated in front of the left-hand edge of a big red-roofed house with two gables (see pic. 38.1). If they cannot be located, a compass bearing on the left-hand edge of the house should suffice. By night stay within the 5°W sector. There is also an approach across the bar farther to the E, a W house in line with the Poundstone Bn at 327°, but this is not recommended except in calm weather near the top of the tide.

The bar is dangerous in strong onshore winds especially against an ebb tide, and has only 0m7 over it, less in some years. The bar should not be attempted under these conditions, or when a swell is running in until there is ample tide. It is here that a lifeboat was lost. The entrance and bar are protected by land from the W and in normal conditions present no difficulties.

Once over the bar continue on the leading line leaving to port the Bass Rock (dries 0m9) off Splat Pt, and to starboard the Wolf Rock (dries 0m6) marked by a G con buoy. As the Blackstone Bn Lt comes abeam to starboard and you come into the W sector of its Q WR Lt alter to leave to port the Poundstone and two Bns off Sandhill Point and proceed on 042° up the middle of the wide fairway.

The front leading Lt is Q W 5m, whilst the rear one is Oc W 4.5s. on a stone column at 45m elevation. They are situated near Scoble Point on the E side of 'The Bag' and lead as far as the port-hand ferry landing Lt F R and anchorage. It is possible to

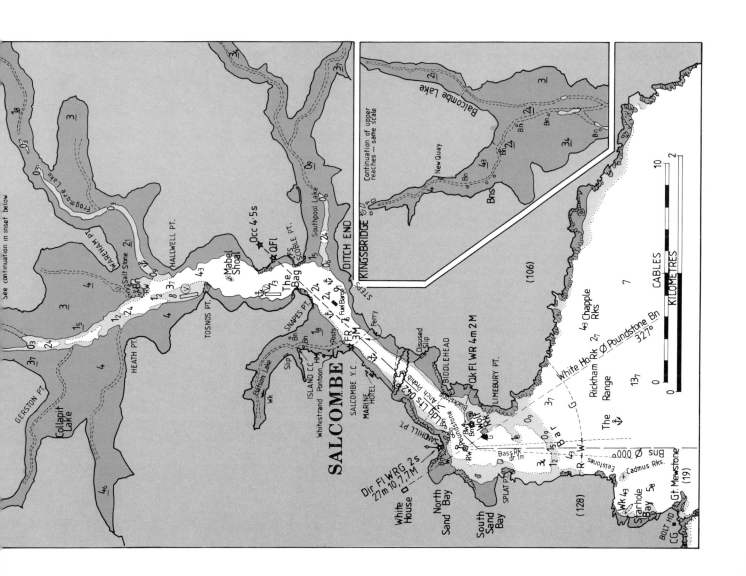

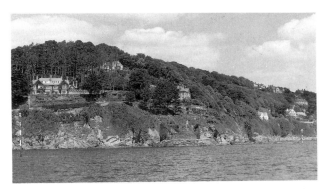

38.1 *The leading beacons nearly in transit with left-hand edge of conspicuous red-roofed house with twin gables. Old Harry beacon on the right. At this point you should come to starboard on to 042° transit for going up-harbour*

continue on the transit to 'The Bag' by bringing the rear Lt just open to the right of the front one when passing Snapes Pt, given sufficient moonlight to avoid the boats on their moorings. The R sector of Blackstone Bn Q covers the Wolf rock on inward passage and shoal water on the eastern bank when departing.

Anchorage and Moorings

(1) *In the range outside* the bar during offshore winds in settled weather.

(2) *Outside in Starehole Bay* in 4m to 6m but avoid the wreck a cable off the NW corner.

(3) Large yachts usually bring up *off the Marine Hotel*, but it can be rough here in strong SW winds.

(4) Off the mud flats between Salcombe and *Snapes Point*.

(5) *Off Ditch End*, on S side of the channel E of Salcombe. Convenient landing here, then short walk to ferry boat landing,

but visitors' moorings now occupy best positions.

(6) *In 'The Bag'*, about ¾ mile NW of Salcombe, clear of many existing moorings. Two sets of visitors' pontoons both on W side of fairway: one just beyond Snapes Pt, the other upstream of Tosnos Pt.

(7) In the pool beyond shallow entrance of *Frogmore Creek* in 1m8.

(8) *Moorings*. Salcombe is well provided with visitors' moorings with large W buoys numbered V1 to V22 situated on each side of the fairway. All are capable of handling at least a 20-ton vessel and three between Scoble Point and Ditch End can accommodate 100-ton ships. These can be used with permission of the HM or from his staff patrolling in launches marked 'Harbour Master', who can also find other moorings for visitors on VHF Ch 16, 14 or 6. He can also be contacted by phone: 054884–3791. Under no circumstances anchor near the fairway in the vicinity of the town.

Creeks   The arms and creeks provide a pretty and interesting cruising area for dinghies and shallow draught boats at HW, but a large-scale chart is desirable.

Southpool Lake, which joins the main channel opposite Salcombe, has uneven depths and the pools are occupied by moorings.

Frogmore Creek, which joins on the E side above Tosnos Pt, also has an uneven bottom with depths ranging from a pool with 1m8 shallowing farther E to 0m3.

The upper reaches of the main channel are marked by RW posts on the mud on the port hand above Gerston Point and are navigable at HW to Kingsbridge.

Facilities   The principal facilities for visitors are centred near Whitestrand Landing Pontoon where yachts can secure for up to 2 hours next to HM's office. Water, diesel oil, petrol and chandlers near by. Fuel barge in fairway (Ch 6 VHF). Water from water boat if bucket hung in rigging. Six boatyards. Grid.

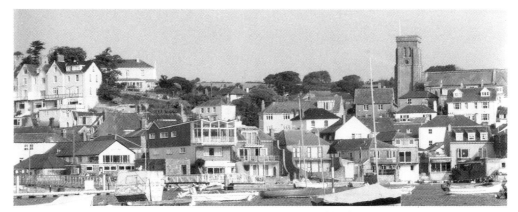

38.2 *Waiting and landing pontoons at Whitestrand. Harbour Office is in front of white-gabled building on the left, immediately alongside walkway to shore (John Robertson)*

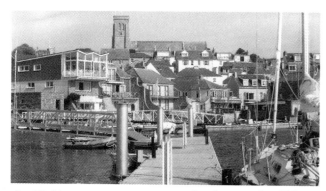

38.3 *Waiting pontoons can accommodate large yachts (John Robertson)*

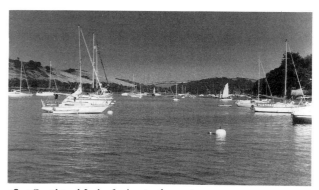

38.4 *Southpool Lake facing to the east*

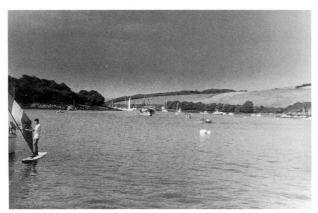

38.5 *Approach to 'The Bag'*

Launching slip 2h. each side HW, and car park, often crowded. Customs House opposite the Salcombe Hotel. Banks, hotels, restaurants and a good range of shops. EC Thurs. Hourly bus service to Kingsbridge. Yacht clubs: Salcombe YC. The Island Cruising Club invites visiting yachtsmen to use its clubhouse at the NE end of Salcombe. Between Salcombe and 'The Bag' use water taxi service – call on Ch 14.

Weather　See Torquay p. 190.
　　　　　BBC forecast area: Plymouth (Portland)
　　　　　BBC Rdo Devon Plymouth on 855kHz.

*39　Hope Cove

Chart: BA 1613; Im C6 (approach only, no detail)

High Water　−05h. 25m. Dover.

THE CHARMING village of INNER HOPE lies in the cove just to the northward of Bolt Tail. It affords fair anchorage for yachts and small ships during winds from NNE to S in depths ranging from 10 to 2m. Run in on a bearing of 110° towards the old Lifeboat House, and anchor before closing the line of the breakwater wall bearing 030°. There are some ledges in the inner cove, and there is a drying harbour for boats formed by a breakwater. Three hotels. Village. EC Thurs. Bus to Kingsbridge (9 miles). Stores. PO.

*40　Yealm River and Newton Ferrers

Charts: BA 95; Im C14

High Water　−05h. 37m. Dover.
Heights above Datum　*Entrance MHWS 5m4. MLWS 0m7. MHWN 4m3. MLWN 2m1.*
　　Depths　*0m4 on the leading line south of the bar with 1m4 just S of the transit, but sands are liable to change; thereafter not less than 2m1 to Yealm Pool.*

THE YEALM is one of the most beautiful but overcrowded harbours on the S Coast. The anchorage is sheltered and the

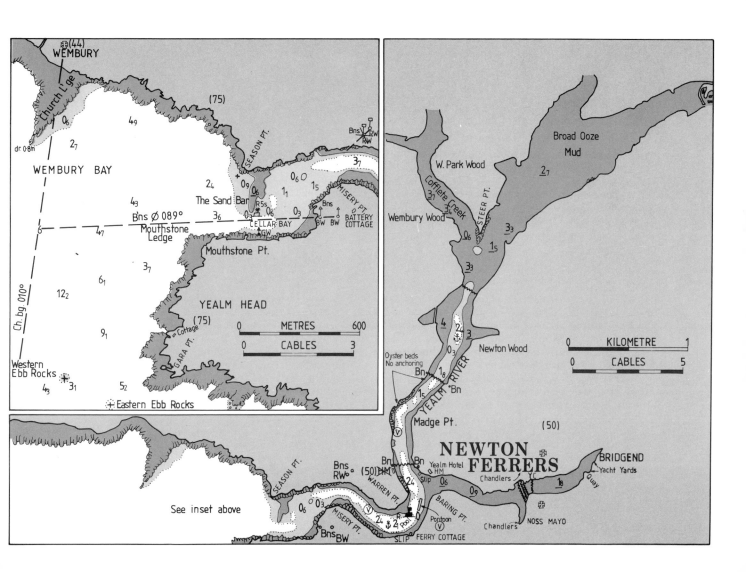

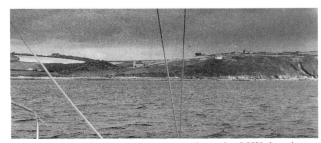

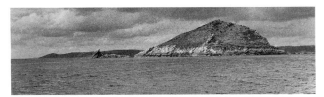

40.1 *The Mewstone from the south-east, with Rame Head in the distance on the left*

entrance easy, except in strong onshore winds. Newton Ferrers is not so well provided with facilities as Salcombe, for example, but no cruise to the West Country would be complete without putting into this secluded river. It is less than 4 miles from Plymouth breakwater.

Approach and Entrance   The entrance is rough in strong onshore winds from the SW, but under normal conditions it is easy enough. The approach is made across Wembury Bay, which lies between Wembury Pt on the N and Yealm Head on the SE. From Wembury head there are rocks and ledges extending ½ mile S towards the conspicuous Great Mewstone Island (59m). On the SW side of the Mewstone lies the little Mewstone Rock (15m) which has an off-lying rock 50m off it awash at LW. Altogether the rocks or shoals extend 2 cables SW of the Mewstone. In this vicinity there are tide rips when the wind is across the stream. A quarter of a mile eastward of the Mewstone lie the Inner (dry 3m0) and Outer Slimers (1m5).

Approaching from the N or W the Mewstone should be rounded at a distance of ¼ mile before standing ENE into Wembury Bay to pick up the leading marks, taking care to leave the dangerous Outer Slimers (dry 1m5) to port.

When the entrance of the river is opened up, a white cottage will be seen between trees near the summit on Misery Point (the inner point on the S side of the river) and below it, above Cellar

40.2 *Approaching the river entrance from the SSW, keeping Wembury church open on starboard bow*

Bay, a pair of leading Bns at 089° each topped by W triangles with a Vert B line. Bring these into line. After leaving Mouthstone Ledges to starboard keep 40m south of the transit, steering near the rocky shore on the starboard hand. In the summer there is a R buoy (Fl 5s.) marking the outer end of the bar. A G Bn with triangular topmark on the south foreshore marks the starboard limit of the channel.

Approaching from the S or eastward keep at least 3 cables off Gara Point to clear the Eastern and Western Ebb rocks (awash). Then come on the leading mark which is the square tower of St Werburgh's Church (about a mile E of Wembury Pt) bearing 010°. The Ebb rocks will be left close to starboard. Hold on until the leading marks in Cellar Bay have been identified. Then alter on to their transit.

The bar lies S of Season Pt with least depth of 0m4 on the transit of the triangle-topped leading marks above Cellar Bay. When about 1½ cables off the lower leading mark, course has to be altered to port to the next leading Bn which will be seen to the NE on the hillside to the right of a clump of trees about 3 cables E of Season Pt. It has a W board with an R Vert line and leads through the first bend in the channel on 047° but an arm of the

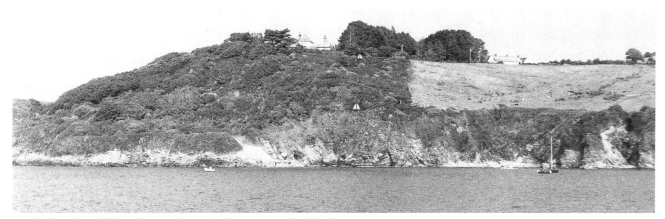

40.3 *Cellar Bay with leading marks on 089° to pass south of the bar*

bar with only 0m6 is close to port. After that the river is clearly defined and it is merely necessary to keep near mid-channel taking care to leave to port the R can buoy on the N side of the Pool. Note from the harbour plan that the deep channel is very narrow (50m) off the eastern extremity of Warren Pt with only 0m3 on its W side and 0m4 on the E.

Above Warren Pt, the Newton Ferrers creek opens out on the E side and becomes Newton Ferrers Arm. It is wide but dries out at LW. The River Yealm itself continues above Warren Pt first in a NNW direction and then bears through N to NE. The bottom is uneven, with depths of 3m4 to 1m8 for over ½ mile, but with shallower patches as far as Shortaflete Creek.

Anchorage and Moorings The Yealm has become so popular that there is now no area left for anchoring in the Pool except in the fairway. The HM can be reached by phone at 0752–872533. Holding ground in parts of the river is poor and yachts should lay out two anchors, which should be buoyed if close to moorings.

(1) *Anchor outside* in settled weather only. SW of Misery Point off Cellar Bay in from 0m3 to 1m2 beyond the junction of leading lines, sheltered from E and S.

(2) Anchor in the pool *W of Warren Point*. Moorings are available on application to the HM, including a trot S of Madge Point where yachts moor fore-and-aft. Anchoring is forbidden on the oyster beds which lie between Madge Point and the next Bns marking a submerged cable, approx 300m farther upstream.

(3) Off *Newton Wood* ½ mile farther up Yealm river there is good anchoring.

(4) On the E side of the fairway round Warren Pt there is a 150-ft pontoon, which can take 25 yachts. You can land at the ferry

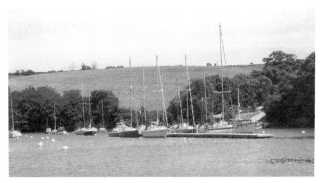

40.4 *Visitors' pontoons on the east side of the river (John Robertson)*

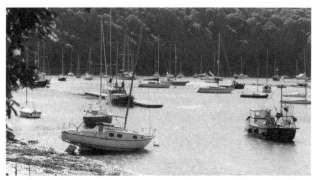

40.5 *Low-water view of visitors' pontoons taken from dinghy landing at Baring Point*

steps at Baring Point.

It is permissible to pick up a vacant mooring, provided you inform the HM without delay. His office is at the Yealm Hotel, which has its own dinghy landing steps.

Facilities   Water at private tap by Ferry cottage near slip, or free at tap on Ferry steps under Yealm Hotel. Stores, chandlery and PO at Newton Ferrers and Noss Mayo, also petrol and oil. EC Thurs. Scrubbing can be arranged. Two boat-builders. Hotels – Old Ship at Noss Mayo is recommended. Yealm YC opposite Noss Mayo. Newton Ferrers Sailing School.

Launching sites:
(1) Slip for launching at Bridgend Quay $2\frac{1}{2}$ h. either side of HW.
(2) At the Brook, Newton Ferrers, same hours.
(3) Also at Riverside road W. $3\frac{1}{2}$ h. either side of HWS or $4\frac{1}{2}$ h. at HWN.

HM at Newton Ferrers. Buses to Plymouth.

Weather   See Plymouth p. 200.

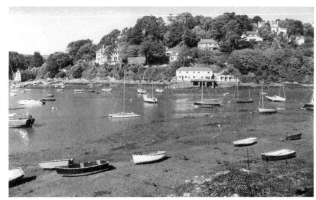

40.6 *Newton Ferrers seen from Baring Point, with Yealm River to the left and approaches to Noss Mayo on right. Prominent building at centre is Yealm Hotel, with Harbour Office adjacent*

41 Plymouth

Charts: BA 30, 1901, 1902, 1967; Im C14; Stan 13

High Water *Breakwater −05h. 49m. Dover.*
Heights above Datum *Devonport: MHWS 5m5. MLWS 0m8. MHWN 4m4. MLWN 2m2.*
Depths *A deep water harbour used by large ships. In the fairway the R. Tamar has least depths of 2m4 as far as Cargreen, 1½ miles above the bridge at Saltash. Thereafter shoal draught boats can continue to Gunnislake, 16 miles from the breakwater, but yachts with masts should watch out for overhead power cables and verify their clearances on chart p. 212. Note cable from Lime Pt at entrance to R. Tavy has only 8m under it at MHWS.*

PLYMOUTH is first and foremost a naval port, the base from which Drake and Hawkins sailed out to plunder Spanish trade in the West Indies. Nowadays about half the active fleet of the Royal Navy, including nuclear attack submarines, is based there and maintained by the Royal Dockyard. Mill Bay docks, familiar to those finishing the Fastnet or assembling for Transatlantic races is now a limited tidal marina associated with a waterside property development. The lock-gates to the inner basin are sealed, and the basin itself is already half reclaimed to provide a

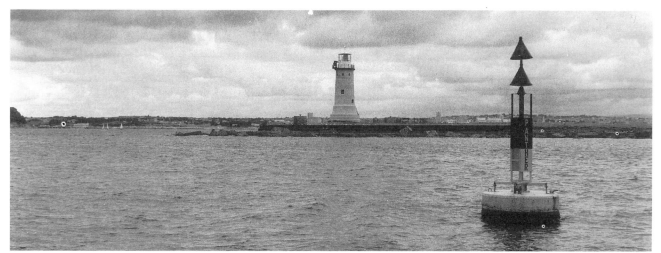

41.1 *Panther N-cardinal buoy and the western entrance to Plymouth Sound*

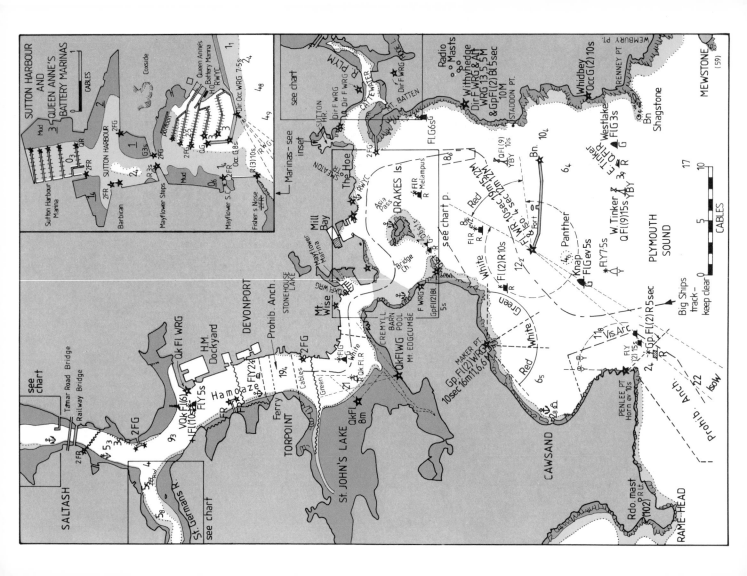

SUTTON HARBOUR
AND
QUEEN ANNE'S
BATTERY MARINAS

CABLES

Coxside

Queen Anne's
Battery Marina
RWYC
Dir Oc WRG 7·5s

Mud

Mayflower Steps
Barbican
Sutton Harbour Marina
Mayflower S.
Fisher's Nose

SUTTON HARBOUR

Marinas – see inset

Radio Masts

PLYM

CATTEWATER
Dir Fl WRG
Dir Fl WRG
SUTTON HBR.
Mt BATTEN
Dir Fl WRG
Fl G6sG

Withyhedge
Dir F WRG & Alt
WRG 13·5M
& GpFl(2)Bl·5sec
10M

Whidbey
OccG(2)10s

STADDON PT.
RENNEY PT.
WEMBURY PT.

MEWSTONE
(59)

Bn.
Shagstone
Westlake
E.Tinker
R Fl G3s
QkFlY 10s
Bn. 10₄

The Hoe
RWYC
SMEATON
Pier
DRAKES Is.
Fl R
R Melampus
Asia Pass

Mill
Bay
Mayflower Marina
Dir WRG
Mt. Wise
Bridge Ch.
GpFl(2)Bl
F WRG

STONEHOUSE
LAKE
Prohib. Anch.
DEVONPORT
QkFl WRG
H.M. Dockyard
2FG

CREMYLL
BARN
POOL
Mt. EDGCUMBE
QkFlWG
Green
QkFlR
White
MAKER PT.
Gp.Fl(2)WRG
10sec 16m11,6,6M

Tamar Road Bridge
Railway Bridge
see chart
SALTASH
St. Germans R.
see chart
2FR

VQkFl(6)
+Fl(10)s
FlY5s
Hamoaze
FlY2s
Ferry
TORPOINT
QkFl
8m

St. JOHN'S LAKE

CAWSAND
PENLEE PT.
Horn 20s
GpFl(2)R5sec
FlY(2)15s
Prohib. Anch.
Isow
Vis Arc

RAME HEAD
Rdo.mast
(102)Fl Lt.

PLYMOUTH SOUND

Fl(2)R10s
R
White
Green
Red
White
Red
Panther
Knap
FlGev5s
FlY7·5s
QFl(9)15s YBY
W.Tinker
QFl(9)15s YBY

Fl WR
10sec
Fort
FlR 8s
R
Red
QFl(9)
10s
YBY

Big Ships
track –
keep clear

CABLES
0   5   10   17

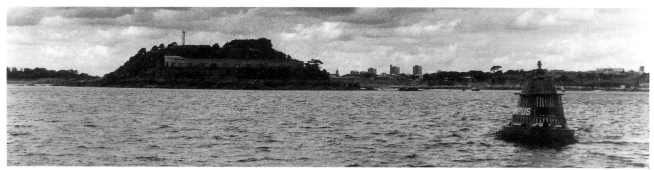

41.2 *Melampus buoy with Drake's Island beyond*

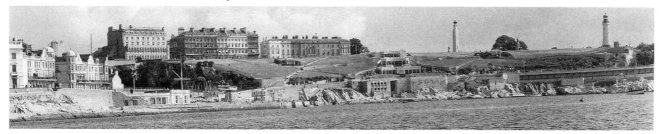

41.3 *The Hoe. To the right are the Naval War Memorial and Smeaton Tower, the original Eddystone lighthouse erected in 1759 and moved here in 1832. It has no light. At left on the water's edge are the former premises of the Royal Western Yacht Club, with flagstaff*

parking area for trucks using the RO/RO ferry to Brittany. There are three other large yacht marinas for those who find anchoring off in 4 sq miles of The Sound a bit remote. It is the finest natural harbour in the English Channel.

Inside the harbour is the R. Tamar running northward above Saltash, which is navigable and sheltered – the clearance under the high-tension wires 4 cables S of Cargreen is 19m at MHWS.

The Tavy joins the Tamar about 1¼ miles above Saltash. This is a pretty river and though yachts cannot pass under the bridge it is navigable by small craft at HW, but note high-tension wires clearance (12m). Below Saltash the St German's (or Lynher) River joins the Hamoaze and extends in a westerly direction. The river is deep for about 2 miles and is navigable. Large-scale charts are desirable for navigating the upper reaches of these

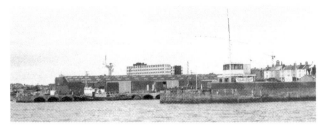

41.4 *Signal station at entrance to Mill Bay docks*

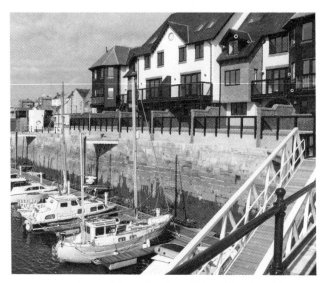

41.5 *New Mill Bay Village Marina. Visitors' berths seldom available*

Creeks. The whole harbour is under the jurisdiction of the Queen's HM and controlled from the Longroom Port Control Station W of Mill Bay docks on Ch 16, 8, 12 or 14 and can be contacted by phone on 0752–663225.

Anchoring is forbidden in any fairway. Keep clear of all warships and other major craft. Full details of Traffic Control signals are in the *Channel Pilot*. The one that matters is a R flag with W diagonal stripe (by day) or RGG Lts: 'No movement in main channel allowed. Small craft keep clear.'

Approach and Entrance Plymouth Sound lies between Penlee Point on the W and Wembury Point (off which lies the Mewstone) on the E. Within the Sound is a long low breakwater in the centre with channels each side of it. The principal approach to the harbour is through the western channel but the eastern channel is equally navigable.

The Eddystone Lighthouse (Fl (2) W 10s. 41m 24M Horn (3) 60s) is situated 10 miles off the entrance: a course of 024° from the lighthouse leads to W breakwater head. From the westward a vessel will first pass Rame Head which appears as an almost conical promontory with the ruins of a chapel at its summit. A mile and a quarter farther is Penlee Point, a low headland with a turreted Bn. Neither is lit. The Draystone rocks (over most of which there is 1m8) extend ¼ mile to the SE of Penlee Point, and are marked by an R can buoy (Fl (2) R 5s.)

A conspic 23m W Tr marks the western end of the breakwater only 1½ miles ahead. Its light is Fl WR 10s. 19m 15M. It has an Iso W4s. Lt 4° either side of 035°, which is a safe course from Draystone buoy to W entrance. Keep in the W sector until passing through the western entrance. Drake's Island lies to the northward, distant 1¼ miles. The main fairway leads NE and is marked on the port hand by the R New Grounds (Fl R 2s.) and Melampus can (Fl R 4s.) buoys towards the famous Plymouth Hoe and thence through the Asia Pass. Yachts need not keep to the big ship fairway and can leave the buoys on the wrong side

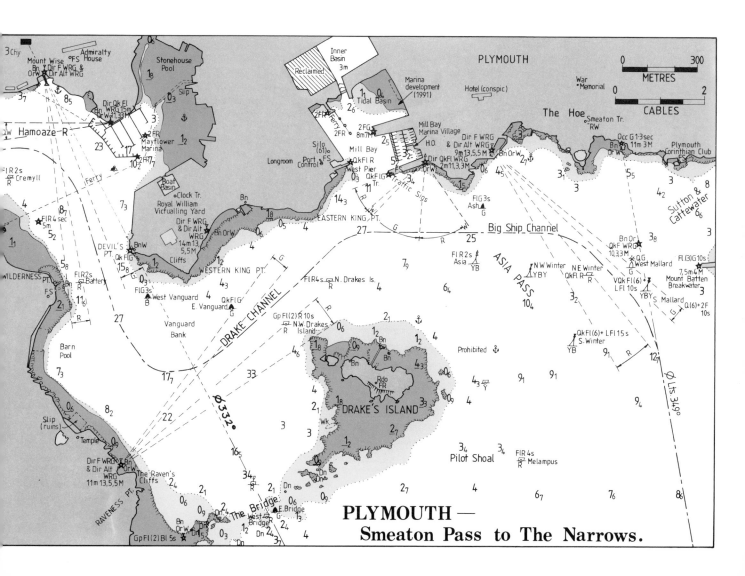

PLYMOUTH —
Smeaton Pass to The Narrows.

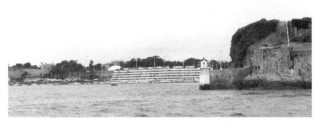

41.6 *Rounding Devil's Point at entrance to Hamoaze River. Mayflower Marina ahead*

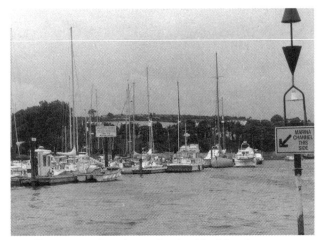

41.7 *Entrance to Stonehouse Creek with visitors' pontoons at far end of Mayflower Marina (John Robertson)*

by reference to the chart (see plan).

There is a short cut with 2m1 to the Hamoaze between Drake's Island and the Mount Edgcumbe shore known as 'The Bridge'. This channel is marked by an R can porthand buoy and G con starboard-hand buoy. As there are underwater obstructions each side of the entrance of the channel steer 332° for it on a transit of Devil's Pt and a conspic house with three chimneys on skyline between the buoys and continue for 150m, until leaving a R buoy very close to port, after which the main Drake Channel is soon entered. The bridge buoys are unlit.

From the eastward the Mewstone (59m) and the rocks SW of it will be left to starboard. Next the Shagstone, off Renney Pt (a nearly square rock 1m2 high marked by a B and O Bn surmounted by a cone), should be given a good berth as the tide may be setting across the rocks between it and the shore. Continue northward passing between the breakwater (unlit Bn at east extremity) and Staddon Point, leaving the coastline to starboard until the channel between Drake's Island and Mount Batten is approached. Here course may be altered to take the Asia pass or the Smeaton Pass or, if bound for the Barbican or Cattewater, hold on to Mount Batten breakwater end (Fl (3) G 10s.) leaving it to starboard and the Mallard Shoal buoy: S cardinal (Q (6) + LF 10s.) and the W Mallard Bn with Or bands (Q WRG) to port. Yachts need not adhere to the main channels as there is depth outside them.

Anchorages and Moorings As Plymouth is a large harbour, the selection of an anchorage depends on wind direction and weather conditions. It is always wise to buoy the anchor.

(1) *Outside*. Cawsand Bay is an excellent anchorage in winds from SW to NW. It has gradually shelving shores and offers good holding ground.

(2) *Off the N side of Drake's Island*. Good holding, but exposed in unsettled weather.

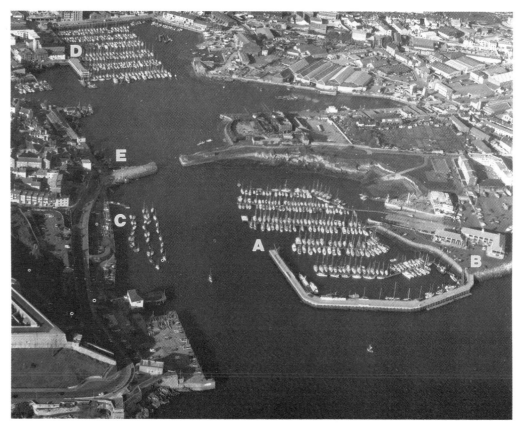

41.8 *(A) Entrance to Queen Anne's Battery Marina (B) Royal Western Yacht Club (C) Mayflower Sailing Club (D) Sutton Harbour Marina and the Barbican (E) The Mayflower Steps*

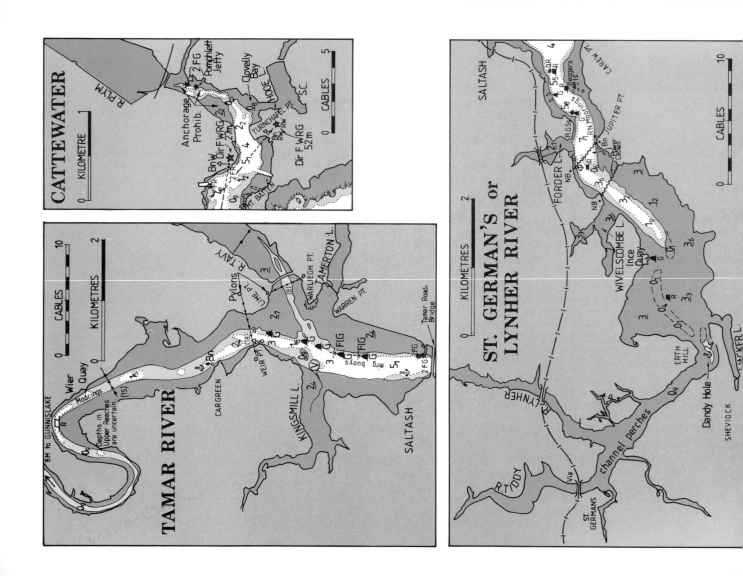

CATTEWATER

KILOMETRE

Anchorage Prohib.

2 FG
Pomphlett Jetty

Clovelly Bay

HOOE L.

R PLYM

Dir F WRG 2m

BnW

2 FR

Turnchapel Pt.
BnW RW RW

Dir F WRG 52m

MT. BATTEN

P.S.C.

CABLES

TAMAR RIVER

CABLES

KILOMETRES

8M to GUNNISLAKE

R
Wier Quay

Moorings

(15)

Depths in Upper Reaches are uncertain

R. TAVY

LIME PT.

Pylons

(181)

Bn

WEIR PT.

WARLEIGH PT.

TAMERTON L.

CARGREEN

KINGSMILL L.

FIG

FIG

mrg buoys

WARREN PT.

Tamar Road Bridge

2 FG

SALTASH

ST. GERMAN'S or LYNHER RIVER

KILOMETRES

CABLES

SALTASH

CAREW PT.

QR

Beggers Is.

RN Moorings

FORDER L.

Bn JUPITER PT.

Pier Cables

NB

WIVELSCOMBE L.
Ince Quay

LYNHER

R. TIDDY

St. GERMANS

Via

channel perches

ERTH HILL

Dandy Hole

SHEVIOCK

R. TACKER L.

(3) Anchor near former R Western YC, in reasonable weather.

(4) *In the Cattewater* (the easterly channel to the north of Mount Batten). Either off the Barbican on eastern side leading to Sutton Pool, or apply to Sutton Harbour Marina on Ch 37, 16 or 12 for a pontoon berth, depths up to 2m1 MLWS, 320 berths. Tel. 0752–664186. The 300-berth Queen Anne's Battery (depths up to 3m0) Ch 37 or tel. 0752–671142 at the entrance to Sutton Harbour, sheltered by its own breakwater (see Harbour plan), has 60 visitors' berths. It is also the new home for the R. Western YC. Water taxi service to the Barbican. Moorings sometimes available on application to the yacht yard in Clovelly Bay, W of Turnchapel Point.

(5) *Anchor in Barn Pool*, which is a bay sheltered from the W by Mount Edgcumbe. The bay is very deep, so work in well towards the shore and let go in about 4m5. Here also buoy the anchor as there is wreckage on bottom. Reverse eddy close inshore.

(6) *Off Cremyll*, near the ferry, but the stream is strong.

(7) *Off Torpoint* in the Hamoaze above the ferry landing and sewer outfall, marked by a noticeboard in 3m0.

(8) *Mayflower Marina* in Stonehouse Pool NE of Cremyll. 250 deepwater berths for craft up to 3m5 draught and 21m length overall; 45 visitors' berths. Contact on Ch 37 or tel. 0752–556633. Access on all tides.

(9) *Mill Bay dock* is now Mill Bay Village Marina with 90 berths and a further 80 planned for 1991. They are strictly for residents, but a call to the Marina Office on 226785 might find one temporarily available.

Tamar River Above Tor Point the river continues wide and deep and there are naval and reserve ships at moorings. Two miles up the river St German's River joins it on the W side, and ¾ mile beyond it is spanned by the high railway bridge and the road suspension bridge at Saltash. The entrance of the River Tavy lies 1¼ miles above the bridge, and here the River Tamar channel is narrow with depths as low as 1m8 near the starboard-hand buoy, with wide expanses of shoal water on both sides. At Weir Point the river is spanned by high-tension cables with a clearance of 19m. At a distance of 1½ cables beyond the Point the best water 1m5 is only about 50 metres wide and a visiting yacht may cross a shoal in only 0m9, but the river deepens to about 4m5 off Cargreen. Above Cargreen the channel requires local knowledge, as the best water is narrow between unmarked mud shoals. High-tension cables (16m clearance) span the river 1¼ miles beyond the village. The pretty upper reaches are navigable by shallow draught boats near HW. Principal anchorages:

(1) *Saltash* on W side below or above the bridge in 6m or more. Anchorage prohibited in vicinity of water mains and cables. Facilities at Saltash.

(2) *Off Cargreen*. Water, facilities and inn.

St German's or Lynher River is entered on the west side of the Tamar nearly ¾ mile S of Saltash bridges, leaving to port an R can Buoy Fl (Q R) marking the flats, the R unlit can marking Beggars Island and to starboard the G con Sand's Acre buoy (Fl G 5s.). It is buoyed as far as Forder Lake off which there is 1m8. Beyond this the bottom is uneven and nearly dries at LAT ½ mile E of Erth Hill except for the Dandy Hole. Above Erth Hill the river is navigable in the dinghy or in shallow draught boats near HW. Principal anchorages:

(1) *Off the bay E of Jupiter Point* but little room clear of Royal Navy moorings.

(2) *SW of Forder Lake* in 1m0 to 3m0.

(3) *In Dandy Hole* in 1m5 to 4m2 on S side of river S of Earth Hill and N of Warren Wood. This anchorage can only be reached at half flood, and soundings should be taken to find the edges of the pool. Two anchors necessary to restrict swinging. No facilities.

River Tavy This shallow river is not available for yachts as it is spanned near the entrance by high-tension lines (8m

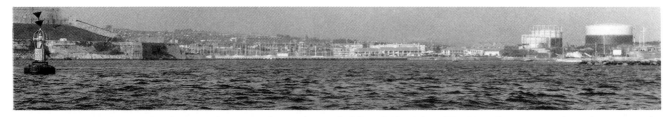

41.9 *Queen Anne's Battery Marina seen from near the eastern end of Royal Citadel on The Hoe with water-taxi service pontoon in the foreground – a short walk from the Barbican*

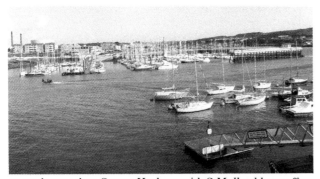

41.10 *Approach to Sutton Harbour with S Mallard buoy off Mountbatten close to port. Queen Anne's Battery Marina in centre of picture (Roger Lean-Vercoe)*

Facilities at Plymouth   Plymouth provides all facilities for anything from a dinghy to a man-of-war and the amenities of a large town and resort area. The marinas offer all services. There are several yacht yards of which Mashford's at Cremyll is best known. Yacht clubs: R. Western YC of England, R. Plymouth Corinthian YC, West Hoe SC, Mayflower SC, Laira SC, Tamar River SC, Saltash SC, Torpoint Mosquito SC, Cawsand Bay SC.

Launching site: the City Council has built a dinghy park alongside the Mayflower SC, Barbican, which will accommodate about 300 dinghies. The RPCYC has also a private slip for club members and there is another at Queen Anne's Battery. Express railway services. Good bus services. Airport.

Weather   BBC shipping forecast area: Plymouth.
Marinecall tel. 0898–500458.
BBC Rdo Plymouth: 855kHz 0605, 0833, 1310, 1733.
Start Point: VHF Ch 25 0803, 2003.
Rdo Plymouth: 1152kHz 0610, 0706, 0750 then ev h. 2103, 2203.
Tel. 0752–402534.

clearance) and by a railway bridge. There are extensive mud flats, but the river is pretty and navigable by dinghy or on the flood by shallow draught low-masted boats.

*42 Looe

Charts: BA 147; Im C6; Stan 13

High Water −05h. 53m. Dover.
Heights above Datum Outside MHWS 5m4. MLWS 0m6.
MHWN 4m3. MLWN 2m0.
Depths Harbour and entrance dry at LW. In anchorage
outside 1m8 to 3m6 about 1 cable E of pierhead.

LOOE lies some 9 miles W of Rame Head and about 8 miles E of
Fowey. The harbour approach and entrance dry at LW; Looe is
not recommended in unsettled weather, as the entrance becomes
dangerous in strong onshore winds. The harbour itself is
unsuitable for any yacht that cannot take the ground or lie
against a quay. The anchorage outside is a good one during
offshore winds and is partially protected from the SW by Looe
Island. Though crowded with visitors in summer months, the
town is a picturesque relic of days when smugglers and Customs
men worked together.

Approach and Entrance Looe is easy to locate because
Looe Island (St George's Island) is conspicuous off the
entrance. The principal danger in the approach from the
westward are the Ranneys Rocks which extend SE and eastward
of Looe Island. To clear them keep the Bn on Gribbin Head
open of the cliffs at Nealand Pt (W of Polperro) until the
pierhead (Oc W R 3s.) bears 305°, then steer for it, staying in the
W sector of the light. A transit of the pierhead and the church
spire in W Looe will suffice by day. Approaching from the E,
keep Looe Island on the port bow until picking up the entrance.
There are tidal rips S of Looe Island and the Ranneys which in
bad weather may be avoided by keeping farther to seaward.
There is no passage suitable for strangers between Looe Island

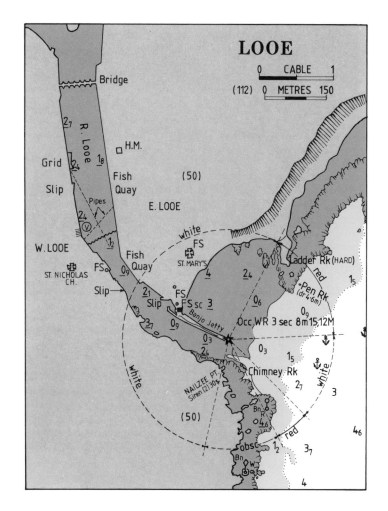

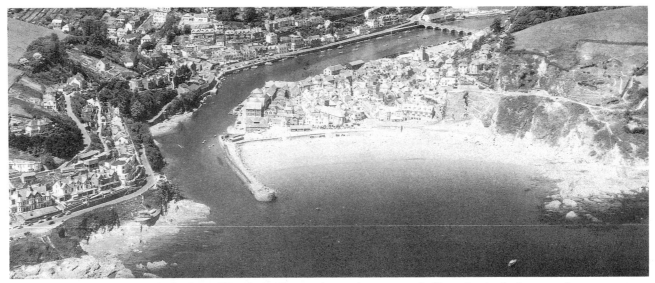

42.1 *Looe River with some yacht berths on West Quay. Best anchorage is to seaward of launches in the foreground*

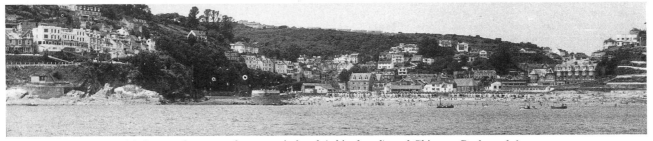

42.2 *Harbour entrance dried out at low water between pierhead (white band) and Chimney Rocks at left*

and the mainland. Once near the harbour entrance, keep clear of the Chimney Rock and other rocks S of the entrance, and of the Pen Rock to the N. See chart for soundings. Just within the harbour entrance it dries 1m4. Wait for sufficient tide. Off E quay there is a reverse eddy on the flood. A R flag is flown from a FS on the pier when conditions in the bay are dangerous for small boats.

Anchorage and Harbour Anchorage in the roadstead is good during settled weather in winds between W and N. There is wash from passenger launches and motor boats, as the roadstead is much used by pleasure boats. To avoid this and because the ebb runs fiercely out of the harbour, anchoring to northward of the scour of the tide from the harbour entrance may be found better, say, with the pierhead bearing about 290°, but keep well clear of the Pen Rock which lies a cable to the NE. Depths range from 1m5 to 3m, or 4m farther seaward. At Neaps it is possible to bring up much closer in.

Within the harbour there are long quays with 3m0 to 4m0 MHWS on the eastern side and 1m8 to 3m3 MHWS on the western. The harbour is often crowded by fishing vessels and other boats, but the HM on the East Quay will direct to a berth on W Looe Quay near the ferry steps. Try Ch 16 or tel. 05036–2839.

Facilities Water at quays or fish market. Fuel and oil. Hotels and restaurants. Many shops. EC Thurs. Boat-builders and repairers and scrubbing. Launching site and car park on E side near FS. Station and bus services. Yacht club: Looe SC.

Weather See Plymouth, p. 220, excluding Start Pt VHF.

*43   Polperro

Charts: BA 148; Im C6

High Water   *−05h. 54m. Dover.*
Heights above Datum   *approx. MHWS 5m4. MLWS 0m6. MHWN 4m3. MLWN 2m0.*
Depths   *Harbour dries out but has 3m3 at MHWS and 1m5 at MHWN. Deepens to 2m5 in anchorage outside.*

POLPERRO ideally recalls the great days when smuggling was its principal occupation. It is now as well suited to being the jewel in the crown of the tourist industry.

It is a small drying harbour 3 miles W of Looe and 5 miles E of Fowey. It lies at the end of an inlet between the cliffs extending about 3 cables in a NNW direction, and is protected by an outer pier and two inner piers between which is the entrance. This is only 9m8 wide and in bad weather closed by a hydraulically-operated harbour gate. Polperro is a fishing village. There is no new chart of the harbour. The plan and soundings are based on a survey by Captains Williams and Bell, R.N., in 1857, coupled with observations by the HM. There appears to have been little alteration during the last 120 years, and trawlermen confirm the soundings have not changed.

Approach and Entrance   Approach should be made from a SE direction when the harbour piers open up. As is shown on the plan, there are rocks extending to the Rannys (dry 0m8) off the headland on the W side of the entrance and there are also rocks at the foot of Spy House Pt on the eastern side. Its Lt (Q WR 30m) has an R sector covering the Rannys. There is deep water up to the entrance of the inlet except for a rocky patch named the E Polca which lies a cable SE of the entrance and has a depth of only 1m0, but can be ignored in good weather with

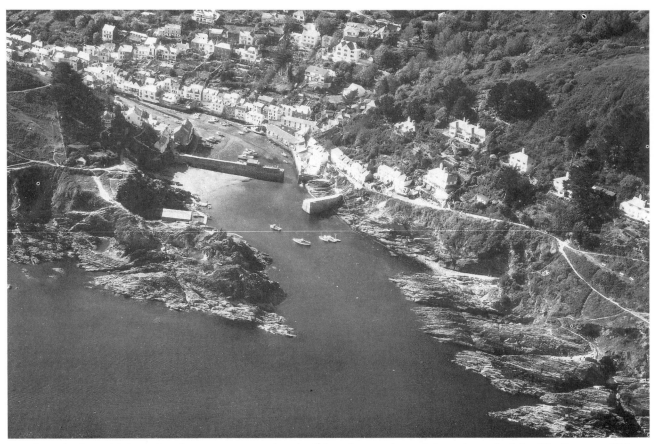

43.1 *Inner harbour dried out, but there are some moorings in sheltered waters beyond the rocks on the left – The Ranneys. Fish quay and Harbour Office are round the bend, top left*

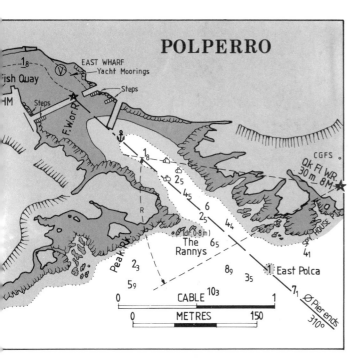

POLPERRO

EAST WHARF — Yacht Moorings

Steps

ish Quay

Steps

CGFS
Qk Fl W.R.
30 m 8M

The Rannys

East Polca

1_8 2_5 4_5 6 2_5 4_4 6_5 4_1

2_3 5_9 8_9 3_5 7_1

0 CABLE 10_3 1

0 METRES 150

Pier ends 310°

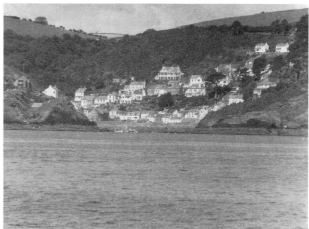

43.2 *Yachts at anchor outside the harbour at low water*

sufficient tide over it. A rocky patch about 30m NE of the Rannys can also be disregarded as this has a depth of 2m5 over it. When the promontory on the W side comes abeam the mid-channel depth is about 4m5 gradually shoaling to 2m5, 1m8 and 0m1 off the outer pier. To approach on a lee shore is dangerous in fresh SE or southerly winds or when a swell is running in.

Once within the entrance the inlet is protected from SW through W to NE.

Keep in mid-channel when within the inlet and approach the harbour entrance leaving the outer pier well to starboard and steering mid-way between the inner piers. The W Pierhead shows a B ball when the harbour is closed (FR by night). When open, it is FG. Strangers should not attempt entry by night. In bad weather the entrance may be closed by hydraulic sluice.

Anchorage and Harbour A few mooring buoys are laid just outside the harbour to pick up while waiting for the tide. There is also just room to anchor although the deep part of channel (2m5) is only about 25m wide. There are moorings inside the harbour but these are of use only to yachts equipped

225

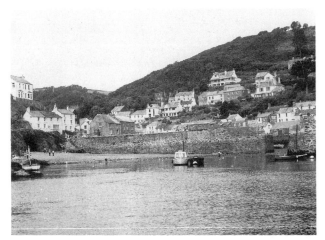

43.3 *Outer and inner breakwaters near low water*

with legs, as the harbour dries out at least 0m6 MLWS. Yachts up to 12m in length are welcome in the harbour and at E Wharf there is a set of visitors' fore-and-aft moorings 18m apart, which dry at LW on hard bottom against wooden posts. Steel ladders to quay.

Facilities   Water at fish market and on the quays. Fuel from Pearce Garage Ltd in village. Several small hotels. Shops. EC Sat, but usually open during summer months. Frequent buses to Looe and occasional to Polruan and Fowey. HM is usually to be found at the Fish Quay on the S side of the inner harbour. Launching site on sloping beach at head of harbour.

Weather   See Plymouth, p. 220, excluding Start Pt. VHF.

44   Fowey

Charts: BA 31; Im C6, Y 52; Stan 13

High Water   −05h. 55m. Dover.
Heights above Datum   *MHWS 5m4. MLWS 0m6. MHWN 4m3. MLWN 2m0.*
Depths   *At least 6m is maintained in the channel from sea to Wiseman Stone.*

FOWEY is an attractive port on the west bank of the R. Fowey estuary, steeped in our maritime history. In the Middle Ages it was the dominant port in the western Channel, relied upon by the monarch of the day to send more ships and crews to support his forays across the Channel than either London or Plymouth. Later its prosperity was sustained by pirates and smugglers. In this century it was the home port of John Stephens and his fast trading schooners, the last commercial sailing fleet in Britain until they called it a day in 1935, having lost eleven schooners to U-boats during the First World War. His ships were fast and wet. In 1900 the 75ft schooner *Isabella* with less than 5ft freeboard made eight round trips to North America in as many months, often taking eleven days for the crossing – with a crew of four. Nowadays it is an attractive port of call for yachtsmen who aren't looking for an alongside berth. It also does a substantial business shipping china clay overseas in large ocean-going ships, loaded upstream either side of Upper Carn Pt.

It is safe to enter in any weather, although it may be necessary to seek a quiet anchorage further up-river when there is a full-blooded SW'ly gale in force. The upper reaches of the river are fun for exploring as far as Loswithiel in a shoal draught boat or dinghy, though they are prone to sudden sharp gusts whistling down the steep cliffs either side or out of openings in the banks.

Approach and Entrance Approaching from the E there is the dangerous Udder Rock (dries 0m6) 3 miles E of the entrance, marked by an unlit YB S-cardinal bell buoy; the only dangers between this rock and the entrance are drying rocks off Pencarrow Hd. Fowey is easy to identify from seaward thanks to the daymark on Gribbin Head, 1¼ miles SW of the entrance. The Gribbin Bn is a RW Tr 25m6 high standing on a 71m headland.

From the westward avoid the Cannis Rock (dries 4m3), some 4 cables SE of Gribbin Head. There are dangers S of the head so far as the Cannis Rock, marked by a YB S-cardinal (Q (6) + LFl ev 10s.) bell buoy. To be safe, keep the cross on Dodman Point open southward of Gwineas Rock.

Once past the Cannis alter course for the entrance, but as there are rocky ledges off the shore W of the entrance give this side a good berth until close to the entrance. Here the only dangers are the Punch Cross ledge on E side, marked by a W Bn

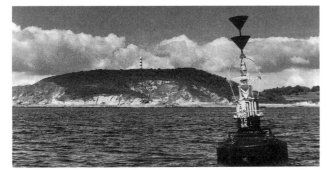

44.1 *Cannis Rock S-cardinal buoy half a mile south-east of Gribbin Head, with its conspicuous red and white tower on the skyline. Fowey lies one and a half miles to the north-east*

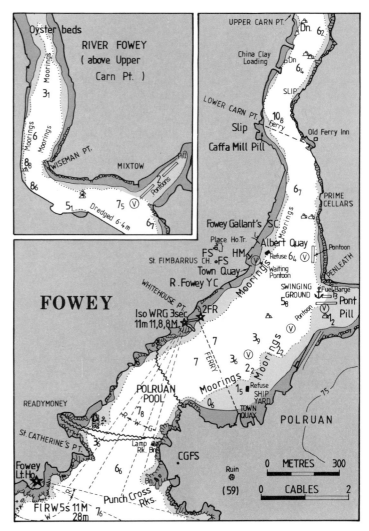

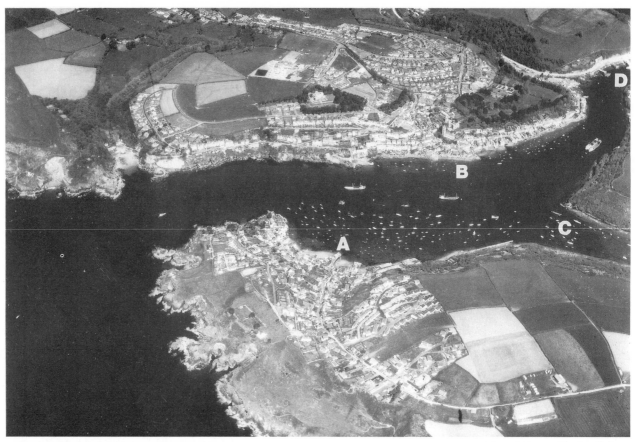

44.2 *(A) Polruan town quay and fuelling point (B) Albert Quay landing with Harbour Master and Royal Fowey Yacht Club near by (C) Pont Pill with two pontoons for visiting yachts (D) car ferry*

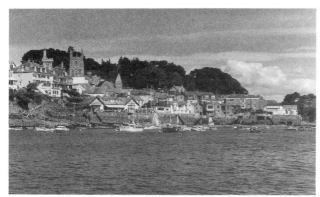

44.3 *Downstream from the landing-point*

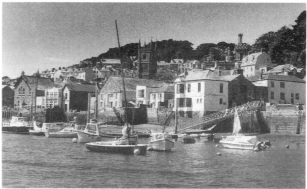

44.4 *Landing at pontoon outside Harbour Office with 2mo alongside. Fresh water available. Maximum stop alongside is 2 hours*

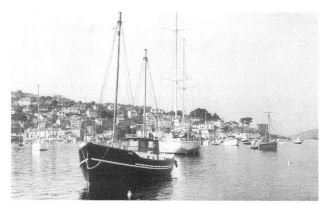

44.5 *Polruan's crowded anchorage facing downstream*

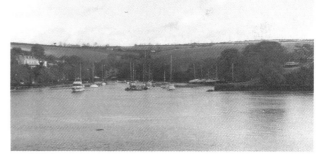

44.6 *Visitors' pontoons at Mixtow Pill opposite the commercial jetty for china clay ships. Served by water-taxis from down-town*

(which should be given a berth of at least 60m) and the Lamp Rock marked with a W Bn nearly a cable beyond it and the Mundy Rocks opposite on the W side. Fowey is a good port to make for in any weather, but the entrance is rough during onshore gales; the seas break heavily in the approach with an ebb tide running against strong southerly winds, but there is no bar to worry about.

Anchorage and Moorings The river and harbour are under the control of the HM. Contact on Ch 12. Tel. 072683–24712. Yachts must not anchor in the fairway, but on the eastern side or in the swinging ground which lies off Pont Pill. All anchor berths only with HM permission. His visitors' moorings are Y or W and marked 'FHC'.

(1) *The R. Fowey YC*, which welcomes visiting yachtsmen, has five moorings on the Polruan side. If one is picked up temporarily the yacht must not be left unattended until application has been made and permission given by the Club; tel. 072683–2245. Yachts may not anchor off the Club.

(2) *The area off Polruan* is crowded with moorings, but it is sometimes possible to find a space out of the fairway clear of moorings. There are chains on the bottom so that anchors must have trip lines and it can be rough on the ebb tide in strong SW winds.

(3) *At Pont Pill* there is a pontoon for visiting yachts and another close by N of Penleath. If anchoring, keep clear of the big ships' swinging ground.

(4) *At Mixtow Pill*, now dredged to 2m0, there are two pontoons each capable of taking 12 yachts. The first one is reserved for visitors. Served by water taxi service (Ch 6).

(5) *In the pool above Wiseman Point*, a secure anchorage, though during gales there are fierce squalls blowing down from the hill. Unfortunately it is so crowded with moorings that it is usually difficult to find space to anchor.

Facilities Landing at Town Quay, Harbour Master's waiting pontoon off Albert Quay (3m5 water) limited to 2 hours' stop, Fowey Gallants SC at Albert Quay, R Fowey YC or Polruan quay. Water obtainable at HM pontoon or Polruan.

Fuel Diesel only from fuel barge next to Pont Pill pontoons. Petrol and diesel from Polruan quay. Otherwise by cans.

Water taxi service (April–September) on Ch 6 available from all pontoons. Polruan ferry will sometimes help. Hotels and good shops – EC Wed. Customs and Lloyds agent. Three yacht or boatyards. Scrubbing by arrangement at Mixtow Pill hard. Yacht clubs: R. Fowey YC and Fowey Gallants Club. Buses. Station at Par 4 miles away. Launching facilities at Caffa Mill car park. Limited facilities at Polruan and at the Bodinnick Ferry Slipway, by arrangement with C. Toms & Sons.

Weather BBC shipping forecast area: Plymouth. Marinecall weather: on 0898-500458 (Lyme Regis to Hartland Pt and NW Brittany).
BBC Rdo Cornwall: 630/657 kHz 0628, 0715, 0743, 0815; w/e 0745, 0843, 0915, 1015, 1045.

*45　Charlestown and Par

Charts: BA 31; Im C6

High Water　−05h. 55m. *Dover.*
Depths　*4m3 at MHWS and 3m0 at the entrances, maintained by dredging inside Par and by the operation of lock-gates at Charlestown. Both outer harbours dry out completely at low tide.*

LYING at the head of St Austell Bay, PAR is primarily occupied in the china clay trade and can only be regarded as a temporary port of refuge, but CHARLESTOWN has a few available along-side berths inside the locked harbour and has the advantage of being only 1½ miles from St Austell. There are plans for its redevelopment and restoration of this charming little harbour.

Approach　No attempt should be made to enter either port except by day in offshore winds or calm. Gribbin Head to the east, with its conspicuous RW daymark (104), and Black Head to the W mark the limits of St Austell Bay. Once inside the bay, **Par** can be seen for miles by reason of its large white sheds and many chimneys and cranes. Run in on a northerly course, leaving the R Bn with W diamond topmark marking Killyvarder Rock a cable to starboard.

Charlestown　will be identified to the E of the houses of St Austell itself. The outer harbour entrance should be approached on a course of 287°, lining up a W patch on the harbour wall with

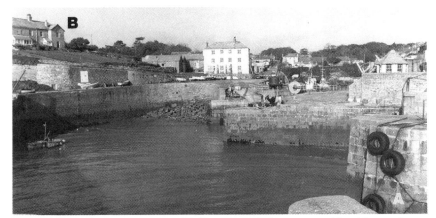

45.1 *(A) Outer harbour entrance (B) Entry transit from seaward is white patch on wall in line with righ-hand edge of cottages. Then turn sharply to starboard to enter the lock-gates at (C) to reach non-tidal harbour*

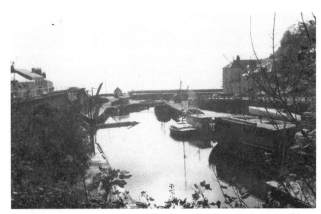

45.2 *Charlestown, the port of St Austell, with a few alongside berths for visitors inside the lock-gates*

the right-hand edge of a row of cottages showing through the pierheads. Once inside, turn to starboard for the lock-gates.

Traffic Signals	Par	Charlestown
Harbour open	—	By night – G Lt
		By day – R ensign
Harbour shut	By night – R Lt	By night – R Lt
	By day – R flag	By day – B shape

Both harbours maintain watch on Ch 16 and 12 (Par) or 14 (Charlestown) when ships are expected (usually one hour either side of HW). Yachts must make prior arrangements to visit either port. If not on VHF, telephone Par (072681) 2282 or St Austell (0726) 3331. Fuel, fresh water and provisions are available. Market town facilities at St Austell.

Weather   See Falmouth, p. 243.

232

*46   Mevagissey

Charts: BA 147; Im C6; Stan 13

High Water · −05h. 55m. Dover.
Heights above Datum   *MHWS 5m4. MLWS 0m7. MHWN 4m3. MLWM 2m0.*
Depths   *2m1 at entrance, 1m5 to 0m9 in the centre of the harbour. The inner dries out from 0m6 to 1m5 and more in some parts.*

MEVAGISSEY is a pretty Cornish fishing village, overwhelmed by tourists in the summer. It has an inner harbour which dries on all low tides, while the outer harbour partially dries. It is well sheltered by the land from prevailing winds from SSW to NW. The northern pier protects it from the N. except in very rough weather, but winds from any easterly direction bring in a swell. It is a bad harbour in strong onshore winds. Fowey (7 miles) or Falmouth (14 miles) are the nearest ports of refuge.

Approach and Entrance   The harbour is situated at the south side of Mevagissey Bay, a mile N of Chapel Pt, 3½ miles N of the preciptious Dodman Point, and 2 miles S of Black Head. The Gwineas (8m high) and Yaw (dries 0m9) rocks lie SW of Chapel Pt, and are marked by an E-cardinal BYB bell buoy (Q (3) ev 10s.) The entrance is easy in moderate weather, but it is only 50m wide, and there are rocks off the northern arm of the pier and a strong backwash when a swell is running. Head for the white LtHo, (8m high Fl (2) 10s.) at the end of the S Pier on a W'ly course, keeping the harbour entrance just open. It should not be attempted at night or in strong onshore winds.

Anchorage   Anchor in outer harbour in 1m5, provided the wind is not onshore. In selecting position anchor clear of the moorings and do not obstruct the fairway, which is in constant

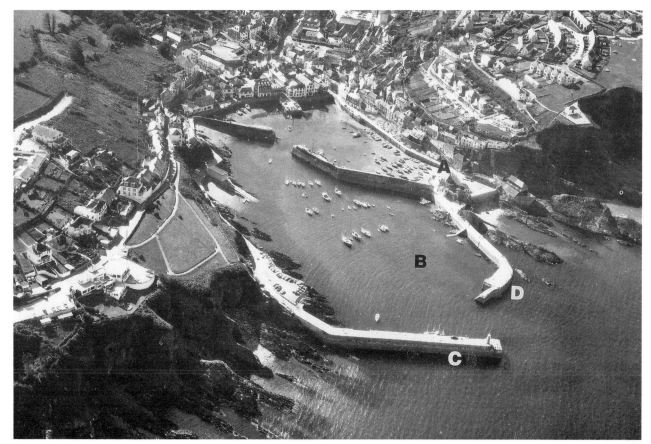

46.1 *(A) Harbour Office (B) Room to anchor in 1m4, but keep clear of fairway (C) South Pier (D) North Pier*

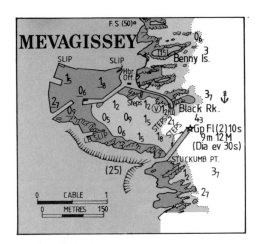

MEVAGISSEY

use by fishing vessels. The best position is on the N side of fairway, but anchor fore and aft to prevent swinging into the fairway. The HM will give directions on Ch 16 or 56. Tel. 0726–842496. With strong easterly winds the outer harbour is untenable for yachts.

Facilities Water at quay. Fuel at Marine Garage at inner harbour. Several small hotels and many shops. EC Mon. or Thurs. but some shops always open. Buses to St Austell, where there is a station. Boat-builder at Mevagissey, also yacht builder at Portmellon, $\frac{1}{2}$ mile southward. Coastguard and storm signals.

Weather See Falmouth. p. 243.

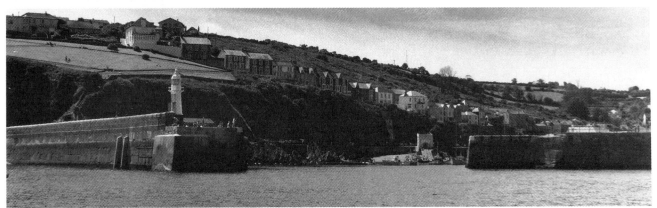

46.2 *Entrance to Mevagissey from the east (John Robertson)*

*47 Portmellon

Chart: BA 148

High Water *−06h. 00m. Dover*

THIS little bay, ½ mile south of Mevagissey, provides a good, though rather narrow, temporary anchorage between the headlands. It is pretty and may be used during offshore winds in settled weather, taking soundings to find best position. There is a good yacht builder (G. P. Mitchell) in the cove; yachts are launched over the sea-wall.

*48 Portscatho

Charts: BA 154; Im Y58

High Water *−06h. 00m. Dover.*

A SMALL drying harbour on the W side of Gerrans Bay, about 3 miles NE of St Anthony Head. It has a street slip suitable for launching boats about 1½ hours each side of HW. During offshore winds and settled weather there is temporary anchorage close to stone pier. Coastguard lookout just N reported Simon le Bon's maxi, *Drum*, capsizing during 1985 Fastnet, leading to a brilliant rescue by RN helicopter from Culdrose.

HM on tel. 087258–616. Harbour dues 5p per ft. PO, pub and village stores.

49 Falmouth

Charts: BA 32, 154; Im Y58; Stan 13

High Water *+06h. 12m. Dover.*
Heights above Datum *MHWS 5m3. MLWS 0m6. MHWN 4m2. MLWN 1m9.*
Depths *The eastern entrance channel is deep and the western over 5m; Black Rock lies between the two and uncovers about half tide. The main channel R. Fal has plenty of water for yachts as far as Maggoty Bank N of Ruan Creek.*

FALMOUTH is a beautiful, natural deepwater harbour, the finest port of refuge west of Plymouth. Its numerous secluded creeks and tributaries, now an infinite source of pleasure to day sailors and cruising people, were once natural delivery points for smugglers. It was an excellent base for pirates to prey on shipping making their landfalls in the West Country and for wreckers to lure them to destruction on the ironbound cliffs near by. Then the locals took to more respectable business as water-couriers, handling mail between Leadenhall Street and great ships making their first or last contact with England during a long voyage, or, when required, delivering mail to or from much farther afield, with inter-city stage coaches linking London. Thus the news of Trafalgar reached the Admiralty. The local newspaper is the *Falmouth Packet* and the Greenbank Hotel still has its rooms named after the captains who relaxed there. 'Falmouth for orders' was a frequent instruction for homeward-bound masters, so the harbour was often full of tall ships during the golden age of sail and much later, while the grain and nitrate trades survived.

Just within the harbour entrance is St Mawes, with clean anchorages in beautiful surroundings, reminiscent of Benodet in

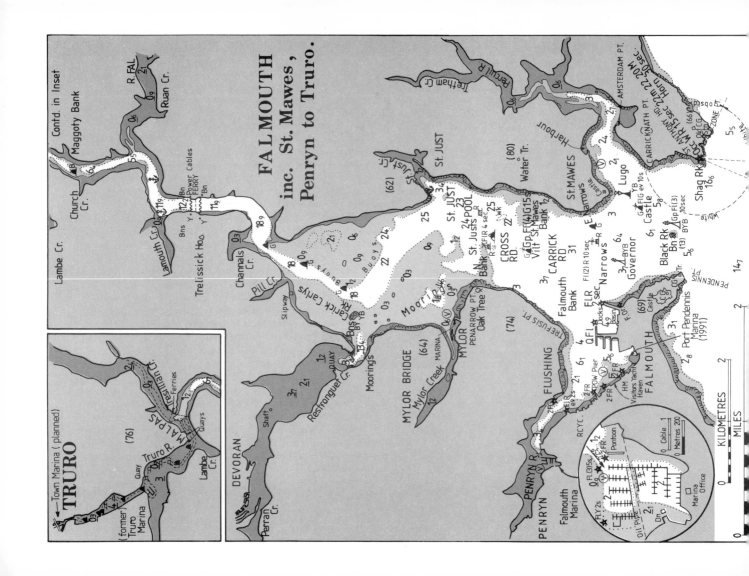

FALMOUTH
inc. St. Mawes,
Penryn to Truro.

R. FAL

Contd. in Inset

Ruan Cr.

Maggoty Bank

Church Cr.

Lamouth Cr.

Power Cables

FERRY

Trelissick Hos

Channals Cr.

Pill Cr.

Slipway

Carrick Carys

Buoys

Moorings

St. JUST

St. Just Cr.

Water Tr.

(80)

St. MAWES

Harbour

St. JUST POOL

St. Just's Bank

CROSS RD.

St. Mawes Bank

Narrows

Castle

CARRICK RD

Falmouth Bank

Governor

Black Rk Bn

Castle

AMSTERDAM PT.

CARRICK NATH PT.

ST. ANTHONY HD.

Oc WR 15s 22sec Horn

Shag Rk

WHITE ZONE

PENDENNIS PT.

Port Pendennis Marina (1991)

Pendennis Castle

FALMOUTH

FLUSHING

TREFUSIS PT.

PENARROW PT.

Oak Tree

MYLOR

MYLOR BRIDGE

Mylor Creek

Restronguet Cr.

DEVORAN

Perran Cr.

Lambe Cr.

PENRYN R.

PENRYN

Falmouth Marina

Truro R.

MALPAS

Tresillian Cr.

Quays

(former) Truro Marina

TRURO

Town Marina (planned)

KILOMETRES

MILES

Marina Office

Pontoon

Cable

Metres 200

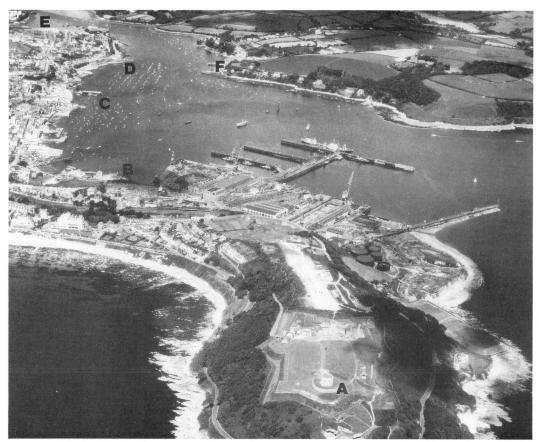

49.1 *(A) Coastguard station on Pendennis Point (B) Pontoons for visiting yachts outside Customs and Harbour Offices, with new Port Pendennis Marina immediately to the right (C) Prince of Wales Pier (D) Greenbank Quay near Royal Cornwall Yacht Club (E) Falmouth Marina (F) Flushing*

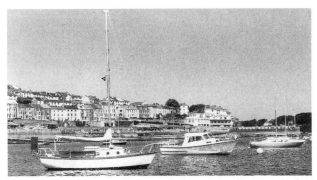

49.2 *At anchor off Royal Cornwall YC, whose slip is on the left. Greenbank Hotel and Quay are to the right*

S Brittany. The River Fal winds its way down from the cathedral town of Truro, past Mylor, a naval dockyard in Tudor times, until joining the sea between Pendennis Castle, the guardian of Falmouth, and St Anthony Head on the St Mawes side.

The commercial docks bear witness to its fluctuating fortunes as a base for world-wide trade, but there is no doubt about the area's recent development as a major yachting centre, thanks partly to better road, rail and air communications, but also to overcrowding in marinas farther E. There is a lot to be said for sailing 100 miles with sheets free to get into the blue waters of Biscay, rather than having to beat 250 miles to Ushant or Land's End from the Solent.

Approach and Entrance The approach to Falmouth from the W or S is safe under the lee of the land in westerly and south-westerly winds after passing the Manacle Rocks. It is also sheltered from the N, though steep seas may be found in the

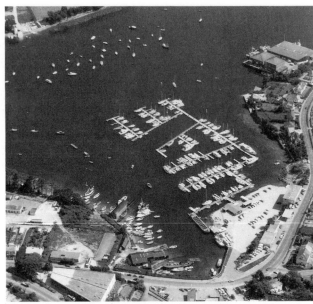

49.3 *Falmouth Marina on the west bank of Penryn River. It now has additional berths (top left) and a buoyed approach channel from the fairway (top right)*

approach during strong winds.

The entrance lies within Falmouth Bay between Pendennis Point on the W and St Anthony Head to the E. It is a deep, easily navigated entrance but can be very rough during onshore gales against an ebb tide.

Approaching from the eastward, give the Dodman Point a berth of about 1½ miles, to clear the overfalls which in bad

238

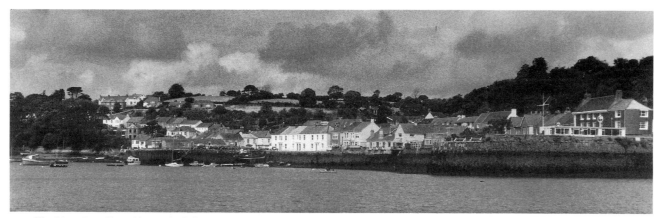

49.4 *Flushing. Landing pier on the left*

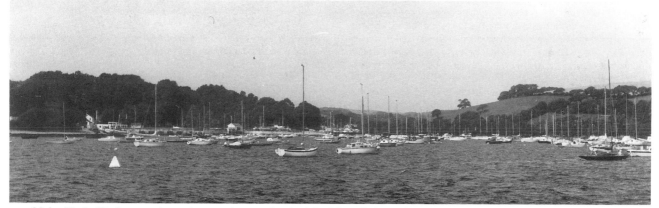

49.5 *Mylor Yacht Harbour and moorings on the west bank of the River Fal, 2 miles from the entrance*

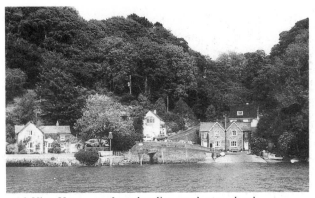

49.6 *King Harry car ferry landing on the east bank*

weather break over the ledges (The Field and The Bellows) some 6 to 7m deep. Also keep well away from Nare Head, for there are dangerous rocks (The Whelps, which dry 4m6) SW of Gull Rock, a very conspicuous islet 38m high, situated just over ½ mile E of Nare Head. Off the next point (Creeb Point), there are patches with only 3m7 to 4m6. Here there are also overfalls in bad weather on these shoals known as 'The Bizzies'. Finally, if rounding St Anthony in very bad weather the overfalls over the rocky patches (with only 7m over them) can be avoided by keeping over a mile offshore, before altering course for the entrance. The lighthouse is a 19m W Tr at the edge of the headland – Oc WR 15s. 20M. horn 30s. Its R sector covers the notorious Manacles.

In the entrance itself the only danger is Black Rock, which uncovers at half tide. The rock is marked by a conspicuous B stone Bn, with globe topmarks, and a BYB buoy (Gp Fl (3) ev 10s.) to its ESE. Black Rock lies a little westward of mid-channel and can be passed on either side, but the main channel is the eastern one.

After leaving Black Rock to port, big ships also leave the W Narrows buoy Gp Fl (2) R 10s. to port and turn to the westward through the 5m8 dredged channel if proceeding to Falmouth docks. Most yachts can steer direct from off Black Rock in a least depth of 3m to join the dredged channel off the end of the Eastern Breakwater Docks Fl R 2s. 20m.

On the eastward side within the entrance lies the entrance to St Mawes Harbour. To enter this leave the G con Castle buoy (Fl G 10s.) to port and steer between this and Carricknath Point (the point on the S of St Mawes River entrance). About 3 cables NW of the Point lies an unlit YB S-cardinal buoy marking Lugo Rock – which is dangerous, as there is only 0m6 over it. Leave it to port.

Anchorage and Moorings

(1) *Outside*: good holding ground, protected from W, suitable for large ships.

(2) *Carrick Roads* (centre of harbour) and beyond. This is used by large vessels, but there is a big swell in southerly gales.

(3) *St Mawes Creek*. In off-shore winds or settled weather there is a delightful anchorage about a cable SE of St Mawes harbour in 1m2 to 2m4. Soundings should be taken as the depths shoal towards the shore and also in the direction of the harbour. Tide is not strong inshore. Drying berths alongside quay in harbour but not much room. Contact HM, tel. 0326–270553. Water, fuel, hotels and shops. EC Thurs. Boat-builders. Ferries to Falmouth. Yacht club: St Mawes SC. In bad weather with onshore winds proceed up-river beyond Amsterdam Point. The area is crowded with moorings but the club has a mooring and there is a possibility of finding a private mooring vacant. Likewise beyond Polvarth Point the Percuil river is full of moorings, so little anchorage is left clear of oyster beds.

(4) *Off Falmouth town*. Contact HM. Ch 16, 12, 13 or 14 or by

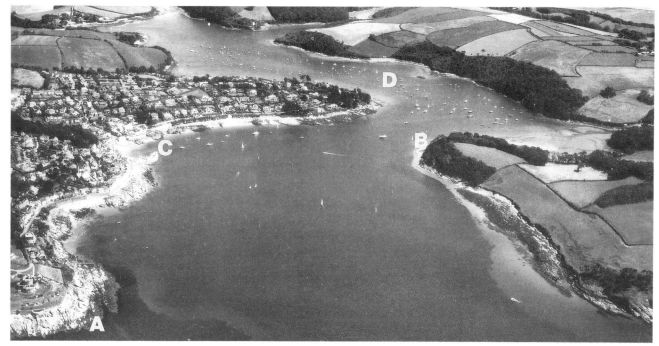

49.7 *(A) Castle Point (B) Amsterdam Point (C) St Mawes Harbour (D) Porthcuel River*

tel. 0326–312285 who may assign a buoy or anchor berth. There are 40 alongside berths up to 12m LOA and 1m8 draught at the Visitors' Yacht Haven right outside the HO. Fuel on tap. The R Cornwall YC has seven visitors' buoys. Contact on Ch 37 or tel. 0326–312126.

(5) *Port Pendennis* is a 60-berth marina associated with a residential development in a basin built to the SW of the commercial docks, due for completion in 1991. Access is governed by a sill at half-tide, with least depth 3m0 inside. It has full facilities. Enquiries on 0326–212002.

(6) *Falmouth Yacht Marina* is ½ mile upstream from Greenbank Quay with 350 berths in 2m0 water, 80 available for visitors. Its

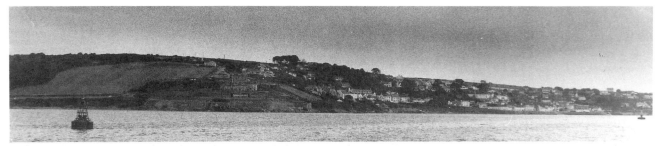

49.8 *Approaching St Mawes from the south-west. Castle buoy is on left. St Mawes S-cardinal beacon to the right of the village*

dredged approach channel on 225° has a buoy (Fl (3) 5s.) to starboard and a Bn with 2F R to port. This leads on to the fuel berth. The pontoon berths to port are private. Call on Ch 37 or tel. 0326–316620. Fuel, chandlery and repairs available. It also has a substantial charter fleet based there.

(7) *Restronguet Creek* on moorings in deep hole W and S of Restronguet Point; avoid shallow patch at the entrance to creek.

(8) *Mylor Yacht Harbour* consists of a small inner dock which dries, and an area NE of it with over 220 swinging moorings and pontoon berths for 35. Contact Ch 37 or tel. 0326–72121. There is about 1m5 LAT in the approach on the leading marks of three prominent trees centre of field to right of Mylor Creek with St Just village dead astern. Facilities including chandlery near inner harbour. Yacht clubs: Mylor YC and Mylor SC.

(9) *St Just*. Anchorage during N and E winds just inside point, also many moorings.

(10) There are numerous anchorages in bays and bights in suitable wind conditions (some of which are mentioned below) but keep clear of oyster beds.

The Upper Reaches The upper reaches and creeks of Falmouth harbour offer interesting day sailing. At HW it is possible to navigate all the way to Truro where there is a quay. There are plans to lock in a 150-berth marina in the town centre with ± 1½ HW access. At LW the river dries above Malpas Pt except for a dredged area 1m short of the town on the W bank where the Truro Marina is located. It is no longer operational.

On the W side of the main Fal channel are Mylor Creek and Restronguet Creek (dries out except for deep hole inside entrance). Yacht club: Restronguet SC. On the E side there is St Just Creek with 3m4 to 1m5 in anchorage and moorings area, but which dries out opposite the church. Ruan Creek, which is the eastern fork of the River Fal joining Truro River, is navigable for a short distance and there is anchorage near the entrance and small craft moorings farther E.

The Penryn River W of Falmouth carries over 2m and is buoyed for ½ mile above Greenbank Quay, as far as Boyers Cellars and the entrance channel to Falmouth Yacht Marina. At HW is navigable up to Penryn where there are quays and facilities.

Facilities at Falmouth Water from N quay, from Flushing quay or (by permission) from the YC. Petrol, oil and diesel from Falmouth Yacht Marina. Excellent shops including chart

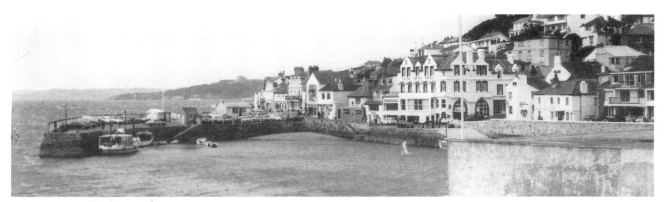

49.9 *St Mawes Harbour and quay*

agents. EC Wed. or Thurs. Many hotels of which the Greenbank is near the YC moorings and anchorage. Yacht builders and repairers. Falmouth Boat Construction Ltd up the Penryn River NW of Flushing, has a fuel pontoon that is accessible at half tide. Chandlery at yard and also at all marinas and Falmouth Chandlers at Penryn. Sailing schools, inshore, offshore and on boards. *Chartering* is big business, bareboat or skippered, sail or power. The largest operator is based on Falmouth Yacht Marina. Customs. Railway station. Buses to all parts. Ferries to Flushing and St Mawes. Yacht clubs: R. Cornwall YC, Flushing SC.

Launching Sites in Falmouth Harbour

(1) *At Falmouth*, Grove Place Dinghy Park, in SW corner of harbour. Launching hard accessible at all times except lowest Spring tides for vessels up to about 7.5m long. Car park immediately adjacent. Changing rooms available at dinghy park. At Falmouth Yacht Marina.

(2) *At St Mawes*, slipway at the harbour, which dries out.

(3) Up the river *at Porthcuel* on E side of river, where road runs to slipway and beach.

(4) *At Mylor* adjacent to the dockyard, car park, and at Mylor Bridge at end of creek, 1 h. each side of HW.

(5) *At Trenewth*, S side of Restronguet Creek, road terminates at hard by SC.

(6) Just west of the entrance of *Pill Creek* ($\frac{3}{4}$ mile NE of Restronguet Creek) slipway and car park.

Weather BBC shipping forecast area: Plymouth.
Marinecall: 0898–500458 (Lyme Regis-Hartland Pt).
BBC Rdo Cornwall: 630/657 kHz 0628, 0715, 0743, 0815; w/e 0745, 0843, 0915, 1015, 1045.
Plymouth weather: 0752–402534.
Rdo Pendennis: Ch 62 at 0803 and 2003.

50   Helford River

Charts: BA 147; Im Y57; Stan 13

High Water   *Entrance +06h. 10m. Dover.*
Heights above Datum   *Entrance MHWS 5m3. MLWS 0m6. MHWN 4m2. MLWN 1m9.*
Depths   *Deep water in the approach; 3m1 on the bar, a mile inside the river. Beyond Navas Creek the river soon shallows and the bottom is uneven.*

HELFORD RIVER is very beautiful, and is one of the favourite yachting harbours of the West Country. The entrance is simple, the depth of water adequate for most small yachts and it is usually possible to get a mooring or find room to anchor.

Helford R. and its various creeks offer a splendid expanse of water at HW for exploring in a dinghy and for picnics.

Approach and Entrance   When coming from Falmouth keep on or E of stern transit of the conspicuous Observatory Tr at Falmouth in line with Pennance Pt until Bosahan Pt (on S side of river) is well open of Mawnan Shear (on north side of entrance). This will clear the dangerous Gedges Rocks, which lie S of Rosemullion Head on the NE of entrance and are marked by a G con buoy Fl G 5s., scheduled for replacement by an E-cardinal buoy.

From the eastward keep in centre of entrance, but before approaching Bosahan Point give a good berth to the Voose rocks, marked by a N-cardinal buoy, some 4 cables eastward of Bosahan Point. Proceed through the 'narrows' and then avoid the shoal marked by a G buoy on the N side of the river opposite Helford Creek.

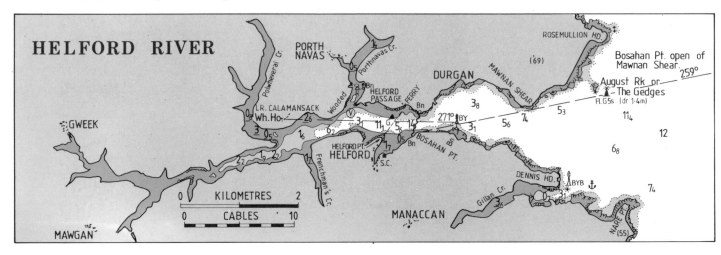

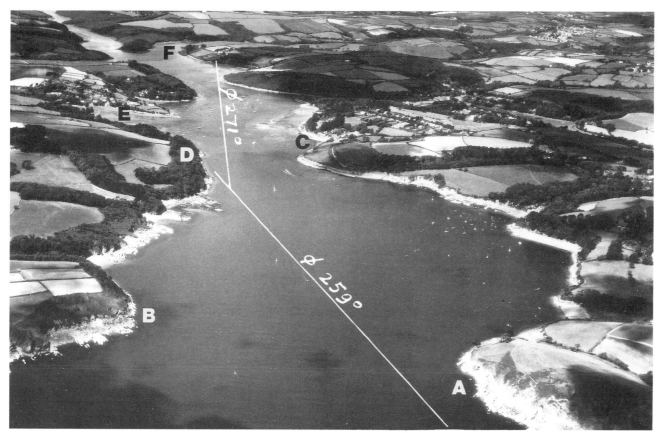

50.1 *(A) Mawnan Shear (B) The Gew (St Anthony) (C) Helford Passage (D) Bosahan Point (E) Helford Village (F) Porth Navas Creek*

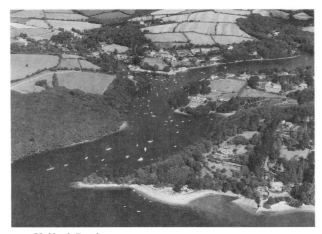

50.2 *Helford Creek*

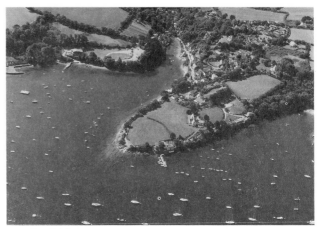

50.3 *Porth Navas*

The leading marks up the river as far as Navas Creek are a white cottage in a group of buildings at Lower Calamansack which should be kept just open on 271° of the wooded point at Lower Calamansack. Entry is not difficult, even if these marks are not located, by keeping on the S side of the river off the ledges and leaving the G buoy, mentioned above, to starboard.

When coming from the W and S keep well clear of Nare Point and Dennis Head.

Anchorage and Moorings

(1) *Off Durgan* clear of moorings in 1m3 to 3m4. Exposed in an easterly.

(2) *Off Helford village* there are excellent moorings off Helford SC and Helford Pt on the W bank. Visitors' moorings are marked by G buoys and marked 'Visitors'. If the HM is not afloat he will be in his kiosk on Helford Pt listening out on Ch 80

or 37 or contactable by phone 0326–280422. Do not anchor in main channel or near cable crossing by Bosahan Pt (see plan). Anchor either to the E of main line of moorings or to the W off Porth Navas creek.

(3) *Navas Creek* on moorings if available, but there may be room to anchor in Abraham's Bosom near the entrance on the E side in 1m5 to 3m1. Keep clear of oyster beds on the W side, marked with B can buoy.

(4) *Gillan Harbour* just W of Nare Pt in 1m4 to 3m1. Only in settled weather. Indifferent holding ground. Avoid sunken rock in middle of the entrance.

Facilities Helford River SC welcome visitors and has excellent facilities. There is a landing-point on the W side of the creek at Helford Pt, where the boatyard has a shop, restaurant, fuel and boats for hire. Helford village has PO, shops, pro-

246

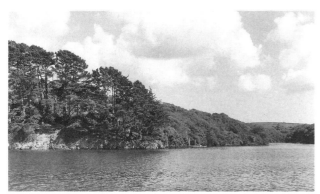

50.4 *Frenchman's Creek*

visions and the thatched Shipwright's Arms. It also has a gourmet restaurant. Ferry from Helford Pt to the Ferry Boat Inn at Helford Passage, which is a hotel and restaurant, where provisions may be bought. Water at Durgan. Buses to Falmouth at the top of the hill at Trebah behind the Inn. Boatyards at Helford and Porth Navas. Launching site by the Inn, which owns the car park.

The club at **Porth Navas** welcomes visitors. It has a bar, restaurant, dinghy landing and limited cranage. It can supply diesel and has the only petrol pump on the Helford R. Minor repairs. Provisions may be bought. Local oysters available from the warehouse at the jetty.

Two miles inland from Helford Passage is **Mawnan Smith** with full shopping facilities, PO, 2-star restaurant and the thatched Red Lion with good bar food. There are three top-class hotels, including the Budock Vean on Porth Navas creek (golf course, swimming pool).

Weather   See Falmouth, p. 243.

*51   Coverack

Chart: BA 777; Im C6, Y57; Stan 13

High Water   +06h. 07m. Dover.
Heights above Datum   *MHWS 5m3. MLWS 0m6 MHWN 4m2. MLWN 1m9.*

COVERACK COVE lies 6 miles NE of the Lizard, between Black Head and Lowland Point. The dangers from the S are The Guthens 2 cables off Chynhalls Point, covered at HW. To the N there are rocks off Lowland Pt, the most dangerous being the Dava rock, 2 cables S of the Pt as it is awash at half tide. To the NE lie the notorious Manacle rocks marked by a BYB E-cardinal bell buoy Q (3) 10s. which must be given a good berth.

On the S side of the cove there is a small harbour, which is formed between the land and the pier, leaving an entrance 21m wide. It dries out completely but at MHWS it has depths of

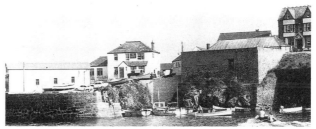

51.1 *Room for only one yacht to dry out alongside the quay. RNLI shed and pub are nearest the slipway. Harbour dries out completely at low water*

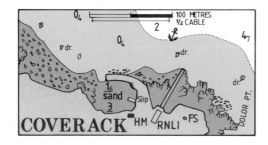

Charts: BA 777; Im C7; Stan 13

High Water *Lizard +05h. 52m. Dover.*
Heights above Datum *Lizard MHWS 5m3. MLWS 0m6.*
MHWN 4m2. MLWN 1m9.

about 3m5. It is crowded with small craft by day but there is a berth at night for one yacht up to 5 tons alongside, preferably twin keeled. It is better to anchor outside, given settled weather and off-shore winds where it is sheltered from the W, but exposed from the E. Consult HM tel. 0326–280593.

Facilities Hotel and shops. EC Tues. Launching site on concrete ramp to firm sand. Water from hotel and fuel (in cans) from the garage.

Weather See Falmouth p. 243.

THIS little harbour lies at the head of Mullion Cove, 1½ miles NW of the Lizard. It is formed by two breakwaters, with a narrow entrance. The harbour dries out and could provide berthing alongside the breakwater or quay, but only in exceptionally settled weather. The cove and harbour are exposed to winds from all westerly directions; even a swell from the W causes a surge within the harbour. Keel boats may not enter and no overnight visitors are allowed inside.

The anchorage in the cove is safer, so long as you remember that it is open to the Atlantic from the W, and should be left immediately if the wind shifts or is forecast to do so. Anchorage can be found in the cove in 3 to 4m with the end of the harbour

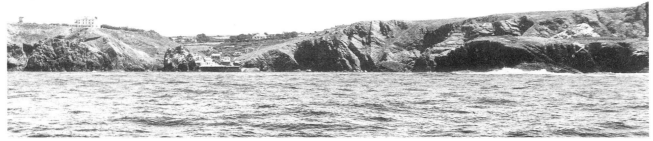

52.1 *Approaching Porth Mellin from WSW. Note conspicuous hotel on skyline left of the harbour*

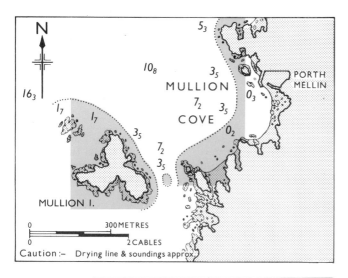

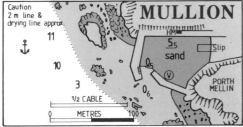

breakwater bearing approximately 080°. The bottom is sand and rock. This anchorage is partly sheltered from the SW by Mullion Island, but not sufficiently to make it a safe anchorage at all times.

There is a café at Port Mullion where some stores may be obtained. Road leads to steep beach where launching possible at HW. Car park. There are shops, a garage and pub at Mullion village, situated at the end of an uphill walk of a mile from the pretty little cove. EC Wed. Launching site on hard beach exposed below ramp.

Weather See Falmouth, p. 243.

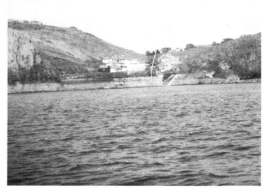

52.2 *Harbour entrance just open at low water*

249

*53 Porthleven

Charts: BA 777; Im C7; Stan 13

High Water   *+05h. 51m. Dover.*
Heights above Datum   *MHWS 5m5. MLWS 0m8. MHWN 4m3. MLWN 2m0.*
Depths   *There is 1m2 in the approach and 2m3 in centre of the entrance NW of pier, but dries out above the lifeboat house.*

PORTHLEVEN is a small fishing harbour situated 8½ miles NW of the Lizard. It may be located by a clock tower, an FS and the white houses in the background, which are conspicuous from afar. The approach and entrance are open to the W, S and SE. The port is now used principally by small fishing vessels. Porthleven is rarely visited by yachts. It provides only drying berths alongside the quay in the inner harbour.

Approach and Entrance   The entrance lies between the Little Trigg rocks off the pierhead on the SE side and the Deazle

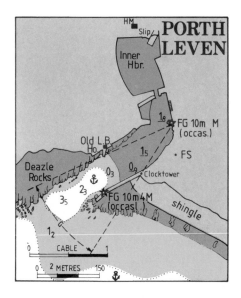

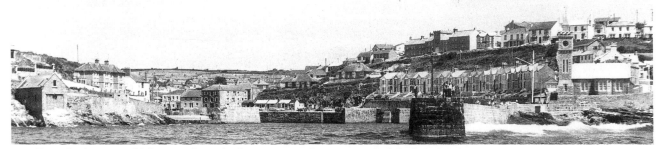

53.1 *Outer harbour near high water. Inner harbour entrance just open to the left of pierhead.*

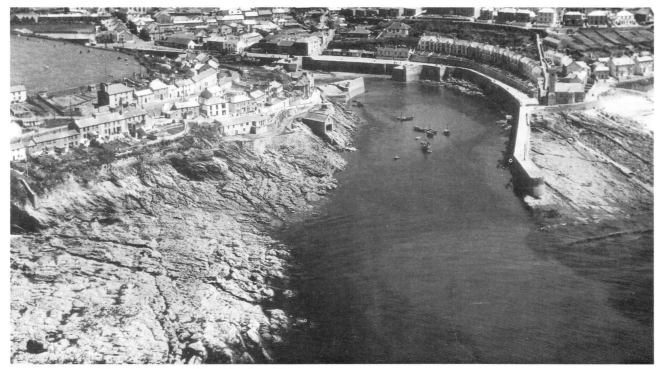

53.2 *Low water, with rocks exposed either side of the fairway*

Rocks on the NW side. It is a difficult entrance because it is only 6om wide and the Deazle Rocks are not marked by buoys or Bns, nor are there clear leading marks to the centre of the entrance. It would be unwise to attempt the entrance without local advice except by day under particularly favourable conditions in off-shore winds. For a visitor to attempt entry by night would be madness.

Approach should be made on a course parallel with the long

inner side of the pier, but about 20m NW of it on the line of soundings 3m5 to 1m5 on the plan. This course crosses a bar formation (which is liable to change) in about 1m2 LAT. At the entrance there are ledges of rock extending about 50m or more off the pier. The entrance lies between these rocks on the E side and the Deazle Rocks on the W. There is 2m3 at the entrance but it soon shoals. Fishing boats occupy moorings in the centre of the outer harbour but most of these nearly dry out at MLWS. When the harbour is closed an R ball is hoisted on the FS at the inner end of the pier.

Lights There is an Occas F G Lt 10m 4M shown when traffic can move; it is about 30m from the pierhead. A second Occas Lt F G on the E side of the harbour near the entrance to the inner harbour shows over an arc 033°–067° when required for craft entering.

Harbour Except near the entrance the outer harbour dries 0m9 to 1m8, and there are rocks fringing the foot of the pier. The inner harbour can be closed with baulks of timber in bad weather. It dries out completely, but by arrangement with the HM (tel. 0326–563042) there are berths alongside the quay where yachts can lie with about 3m at MHWS in the deepest berth.

Facilities Water, fuel and some stores. EC Wed. Boat-builders. Two small hotels. Good bus service to Penzance and Falmouth. Launching sites: trailed boats of any size from ramp, slipway at the head of the inner harbour for launching small craft by hand near HW.

Weather See Falmouth, p. 243.

*54   St Michael's Mount and Marazion

Charts: BA 2345; Stan 13

High Water +05h. 50m. Dover.
Heights above Datum *MHWS 5m6. MLWS 0m8. MHWN 4m4. MLWN 2m0.*
Depths *The harbour dries out but there is about 3m3 at MHWS.*

ST MICHAEL'S MOUNT, with its castle, is one of the most striking landmarks in the English Channel. From AD25, when it was used by Roman and Greek merchants as a base for tin trading, its long and varied history is of great interest. It is now National Trust property – well worth sailing there, or you can walk out from the mainland at LW. There is a small drying harbour at the N end between two piers and there is anchorage to the westward of the entrance.

Approach and Entrance Approach may be made from the direction of the Gear Rock Bn off Penzance steering on the line to the N end of the harbour breakwater at 074° keeping in the W sector of Penzance S Pierhead Lt although it should not be attempted at night. The principal dangers in the approach are the Hogus Rocks to the NW of the harbour, and the unmarked Outer Penzeath Rock, with 1m5 over it, about 3 cables WSW of the Hogus Rocks. These dangers are left to port. Nearly a cable SSW of the Mount lies the Maltman Rock which dries 0m9, a danger only if approaching from S or SE. The various rocks have no Bns to mark them. Kind weather, a good compass and some local knowledge are desirable.

The approach gradually shelves from 8m to 2m a cable W of

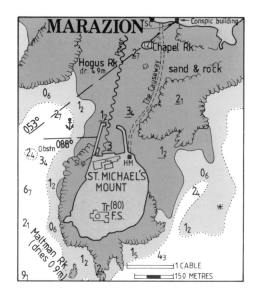

the entrance. Depths then rapidly fall and the bottom dries out northward of the W pier. Do not leave the pier more than $\frac{1}{2}$ cable to starboard as the Hogus Rocks lie only a cable N of it. Then enter on sufficient tide.

Alternatively, approach may be made from the S. Keep well away from the rocks extending S of the Mount. Then follow up the W side at a distance of about 1 cable, but note a rock (2m1 over it) and an obstruction (2m4 over it), dangerous in a bad sea or swell. When the pierhead bears 060° alter towards the anchorage with Chapel Rock bearing 053° in the transit with a conspicuous building or, with sufficient tide, steer direct for the pierhead and enter.

Harbour and Anchorage There is a pleasant anchorage in 2m7 about a cable W of the northern end of the W pier, which can be used in settled weather sheltered from N through E to SE. The entrance between the piers is 30m wide and the harbour dries from 1m5 to 3m0. The HM will direct a visiting yacht to a drying berth, usually alongside a ladder on the W quay; the E quay is used by ferries and launches.

Facilities There are no facilities on the island except water and a café (open Mon.–Fri. in summer months), which supplies some provisions, but all facilities are available at Marazion, $\frac{1}{2}$ mile to the northward. This can be reached across the causeway at LW or by dinghy or ferry at HW. Water, fuel, hotels, banks, shops. EC Wed., but some shops open on all days. Yacht club: Mount's Bay SC. Facilities for dinghy racing. Launching site: at the west end of Marazion on beach, with car park and garage adjacent. Frequent bus services to Penzance less than 3 miles to the W.

Weather See Penzance, p. 256.

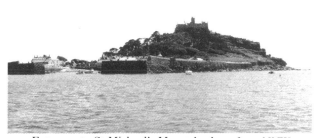

54.1 *Entrance to St Michael's Mount harbour from NNW (Rober Lean-Vercoe)*

*55 Penzance

Charts: BA 2345; Im C7; Stan 13

High Water *+05h. 50m. Dover.*
Heights above Datum *MHWS 5m6. MLWS 0m8. MHWN 4m4. MLWN 2m0.*
Depths *There is about 1m8 close to the seaward end of the S pier. Thereafter the outer harbour dries out completely, except close alongside the S pier where the depth outside the locks is 0m6. The wet dock has at least 4m3. The lock gates are open 2h. before to 1h. after HW.*

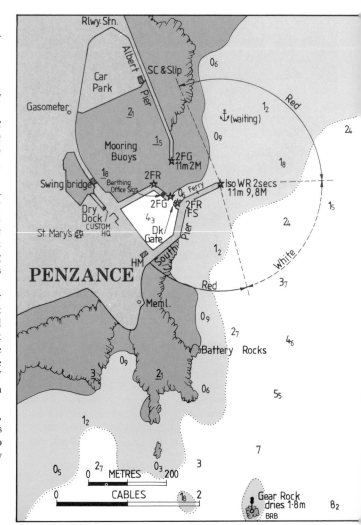

PENZANCE is a commercial harbour but it is also frequently used by yachts as the westernmost port offering shelter in bad weather. It is also a useful port of departure for Ireland and the Scillies. In strong winds from the S and especially from the SE it is dangerous to run for shelter at Penzance owing to the shoaling water in the approach. Mount's Bay is very exposed to winds from these quarters.

Approach and Entrance Penzance lies in the NW corner of Mount's Bay some 15½ miles NW of Lizard Point. A yacht coming from the eastward should keep 2 to 3 miles off the Lizard in rough weather (see Passage Data) or in a fresh wind against the tide, to avoid the overfalls and should shape a course outside the Boa shoal (3 miles W of the Lizard). Farther into Penzance Bay there are shoals S of Cudden Point which are clear once W of the transit of the Tr on St Michael's Mount and Ludgvan church on high ground 1 mile inland on 340°.

Coming from the westward, after passing the Runnel Stone, follow up the coast keeping a mile offshore as far as St Clement's Island outside Mousehole. Leaving the island about 2 cables to port make good 020° leaving Low Lee BYB east cardinal buoy

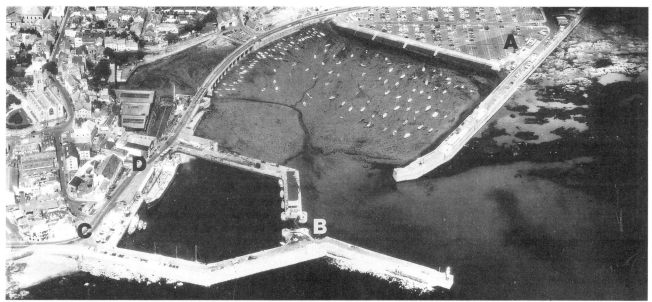

55.1 *(A) Penzance Sailing Club and car park (B) Lock-gates and traffic signals (C) Harbour Office (D) Customs*

(Q (3) 10s.) to port. Alter when Penzance S pierhead (Iso WR 2s. 11m 9M) bears 350° keeping in W sector. Give a good berth to Gear Rock ½ mile S of the pier (which is marked by an unlit B Bn with cage topmark) and to the Battery Rocks to SW of the pier. Then round in towards the pierheads. Note that at LW Springs there is only about 1m8 E of the S pier and see 'Depths' for water within harbour. Four cables NE of the entrance lie the Cressar Rocks marked by a BW Bn. Tidal streams off the entrance are weak.

Berthing One of the HM's staff at the dock-gate may direct yachts to a berth. Or contact on VHF Ch 16 or 12. Tel. 0736–07415 or 66113. The large outer harbour on the N side dries out. Here there are many moorings for dinghies and small craft, which can take the bottom at LW. Keel yachts can dry out alongside the Albert Pier, which is the safer location outside the basin; or afloat on the Quay, subject to the prior rights of the ferry. It is far better to enter the inner basin, where there is usually about 4m2 of water. The gates open from 2h. before HW

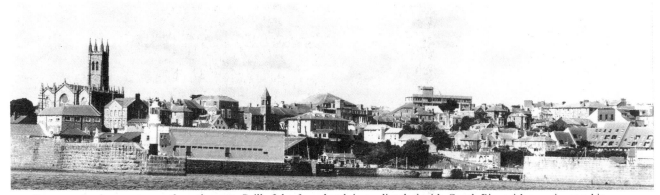

55.2 *Penzance harbour entrance from the east. Scilly Isles ferry berth immediately inside South Pier with prominent white lighthouse with black base. Lock-gates to wet dock and traffic signals are under church tower (Roger Lean-Vercoe)*

to HW. In strong southerly gales the seas break over the S pier of the basin, so the N pier is the better for shelter, although here there is often coal dust.

Waiting for tide, anchor outside about 2 cables E of Albert Pier, weather permitting. Outgoing commercial traffic heads SSE from the pierhead. Keep well clear at all times. The state of Lock Gates is signalled on N side of entrance:

	Day (shapes)		Night (lights)
	B ●		R ●
Gate shut	B ●		G ○
Gate open	B ●	B ●	R ●
			R ●

Local info on VHF Ch 12 at 0910 Mon–Sat covers weather, shipping movements, lock times, warnings.

Facilities   Heads and showers at Berthing Office. Water on all quays. Customs. Two boatyards; scrubbing at hard in outer harbour. Fuel in SW corner of locked basin; chandlery and sailmaker in the town. Many hotels, restaurants, shops of all kinds. EC Wed. Yacht club: Penzance SC. Launching site: dinghies may use the slipway at the outer harbour approximately from 3½ hours before to 3½ hours after HW. Station and buses to all districts. Passenger ferry and helicopter service to Scilly Isles.

Weather   BBC forecast area: Plymouth.
Marinecall tel: 0898–500458.
BBC Rdo Cornwall 630/657 kHz 0628, 0715, 0743, 0815.
Land's End Rdo – Ch 27 or 88 at 0803, 2003.

56 Newlyn

Charts: BA 2345; Im C7; Stan 13

High Water +05h. 50m. Dover.
Heights above Datum MHWS 5m6. MLWS 0m8. MHWN 4m4. MLWN 2m0.
Depths *The entrance has been dredged to 3m9 and to a least depth of 2m0 on both sides of the new quay, which divides the harbour in two. A coaster drawing 3m3 can lie alongside the N pier. Either side of the newly-dredged channel the harbour shallows progressively farther to the NW with 1m8 at the third tier and drying at the end.*

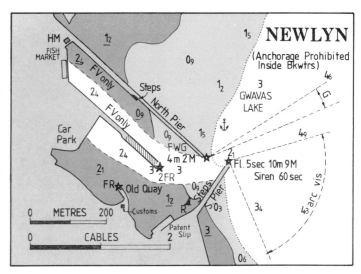

NEWLYN is a sheltered commercial fishing port which offers a muted welcome and few berths to visiting yachts. Southerly and SE winds can bring a heavy swell outside, and the approach would be downright dangerous in a SE gale. It is not normally comfortable or convenient for yachts, especially if not equipped with legs, as it is a busy fishing port with limited room to lie afloat alongside. It is prohibited to anchor anywhere in the harbour. The HM always endeavours to find a place for a visiting yacht, but this is difficult during the season in June, July and August. Then the harbour has to accommodate many fishing vessels from elsewhere in addition to its own fleet. The S pier has 3m9 at its extremity, but should not be used by yachts as it is reserved for commercial vessels.

The best way of visiting Newlyn in offshore winds is to anchor outside in Gwavas Lake and enter by dinghy.

Approach and Entrance Coming from any direction follow the instructions given for Penzance, but alter course for Newlyn when the harbour entrance bears 270°, distant about ¾ mile. Enter between the pierheads; N pier FWG 4m 2M.

S pier Fl 5s. 10m 9M with siren 60s. A small R spar buoy will be seen ahead. This marks the end of a slipway, and course should be altered to starboard to leave the buoy to port. The W side of the harbour dries out, but there is a dredged channel with a least depth of 2m0 parallel with the new pier to within 35m of the inshore end of the Old Quay.

Anchorage and Harbour

(1) *Outside* in Gwavas Lake to the NE of North Pier, clear of the fairway in 2m1, or more farther seaward. Good holding ground and well sheltered from offshore winds from SW, through W to NW.

(2) *Alongside* outer half of N Pier or abreast of other vessels, but apply to HM for berth least inconvenienced by movements of

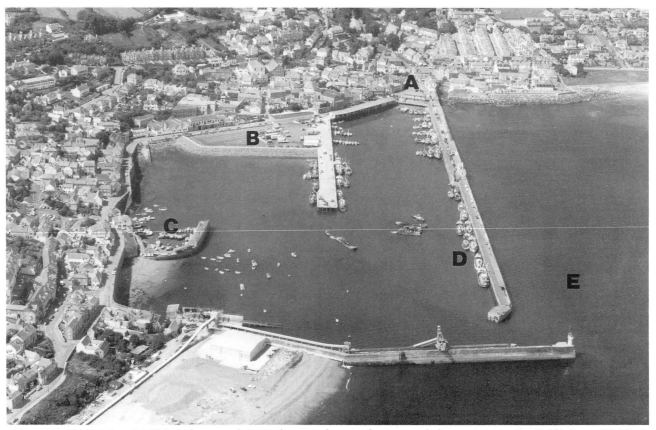

56.1 *(A) Harbour Office (B) Fish dock area – the quay in centre has now been extended 90m to seaward (C) Old Quay (D) North Pier, where yachts may lie alongside, but fishing vessels have priority (E) Safe anchorage in Gwavas Lake*

fishing vessels. Contact the HM on Ch 16 or tel. 0736–62523. The best water is 3m3 at the outer end but the berths are in frequent use by big fishing vessels. A cable from the entrance the depth alongside N Pier is 0m9 LAT +0m8 at MLWS, +2m0 at MLWN. Legs are necessary when not alongside, as no room elsewhere to lie afloat. Owing to the large number of fishing vessels based at the port, visiting yachts must keep sufficient crew on board to move if requested by fishing boats. When the fishing fleet returns through stress of weather, all berths at Newlyn may be required, and yachts are asked to seek shelter at Penzance.

Facilities Water by hydrants at all berths. Diesel oil hydrants and petrol at Ridges on the quay. Customs House. Two ship and yacht repairers, J. Peak & Son and H. N. Peak. Slipway up to 27m4 keel, 6m4 draught available on application to HM.

Three small hotels. Shops and chandlers. EC Wed. Frequent buses to Penzance and elsewhere. Station at Penzance. Launching sites: by arrangement with HM only.

Weather See Penzance, p. 256.

*57 Mousehole

Charts: BA 2345; Im C7; Stan 13

High Water *+05h. 50m. Dover.*
Heights above Datum *MHWS 5m6. MLWS 0m8. MHWN 4m3. MLWN 2m0.*
Depths *Dries out at LW. At MHWS there is about 3m8 and MHWN about 2m6. Bottom gravel on rock.*

MOUSEHOLE HARBOUR is a small picturesque drying harbour formed by two breakwaters leaving an entrance only 11m wide. It is well protected except in strong winds between NE and SE. The entrance may be closed with baulks of timber during strong onshore winds and usually remains shut in mid-winter. In 1981 all eight of the local lifeboat crew were lost in attempting to save

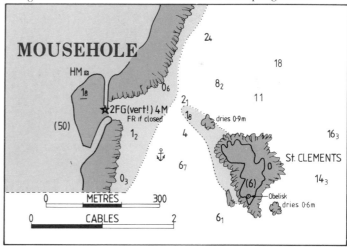

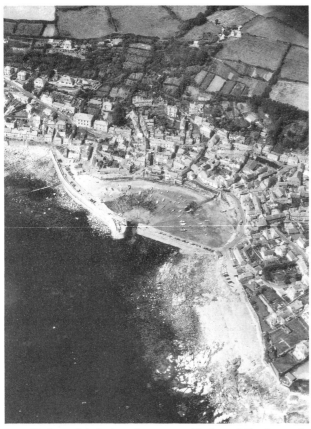

57.1 *Harbour dried out at low water. Harbour Office located at right-hand side of harbour*

a coaster driven on to the rocks just 3 miles away to the SW.

Approach and Entrance Mousehole is situated 1¼ miles S of Newlyn and lies west of the small St Clement's Island, which makes it easy to locate. St Clement's Island is fringed with rocks as shown on the plan; the easiest approach to the harbour is from the southward, following parallel with the line of the Cornish coast to port, and passing rather west of midway between the shore and St Clement's Island. Once the middle of the island is abeam the water between the island and the harbour is clear of dangers, apart from rocks fringing the seaward sides of the breakwaters. Depths in the approach vary from 6m7 when St Clement's Island is abeam down to about 0m5 off the entrance, where final approach should be made when the centre bears 270°, distant ½ cable. The N pierhead shows 2 F G Vert from an R metal column. These Lts replaced by F R when entrance is forbidden.

Harbour and Anchorage Yachts dry out alongside the inner sides of the breakwaters; the deepest berths are near the entrance. The HM will give instructions for berthing, but the harbour is often so crowded that it is difficult to get alongside. The HM's telephone is 0736–731511. The anchorage outside provides good holding ground. It is sheltered by the land from N and W and St Clement's Island provides partial protection from light E winds, but it is open to S and SE, which are dangerous quarters in unsettled weather. Even with westerly winds there is sometimes swell entering the anchorage from the S. Take soundings to find best position to anchor, approximately midway between the S breakwater and the middle of the island.

Facilities Water and petrol. Three small hotels, several shops. The Lobster Pot Restaurant and the Ship Inn draw visitors from afar. EC Wed. Launching site: slipway in harbour. Car park near by. Buses to Newlyn and Penzance.

Weather See Penzance, p. 256.

58 Isles of Scilly

Charts: BA34 (Im C7 – St Mary's and SE approach only)

High Water *(St Mary's Pool)* + 05h. 52m. Dover.
Heights above Datum *MHWS 5m7. MLWS 0m7. MHWN 4m3. MLWN 2m0.*
Depths *Up to 2m1 in St Mary's Pool, 2m4 to 11m0 in anchorage NW of New Grimsby harbour (Tresco) or 15m0 in Crow Sound and St Mary's Sound.*

THESE islands – some forty-seven of them – have a special charm of their own; they are an eclectic of ingredients from England, Scotland, Brittany and the tropics. Historically the locals have been described as smugglers turned gardeners. They may also have derived some benefit from the steady parade of ships piling up on their rocks. The steadfastness of their lifeboatmen is legendary, never more so than during the 1979 Fastnet Race.

Only five islands are inhabited, each so different from the others – St Mary's, Tresco, St Martin's, Bryher and St Agnes; of these St Mary's is the biggest with Hugh Town built around the harbour as its 'capital'.

Any yacht exploring these islands should not do so without a splendid little paperback guide obtainable locally: *A Yachtsman's Guide to Scilly*, by Norm. The charm of this archipelago may lull the navigator into a false sense of security, as there are many hidden dangers in the form of pinnacle rocks with strong tidal eddies around them. Local knowledge is desirable if any intricate passages between the smaller islands are contemplated. Here only the safest four, of the six, approach channels to St Mary's Road will be described.

Off-lying Dangers These are numerous and clearly marked on the Admiralty Chart. All rise suddenly from deep water; mentioned here – only because of their isolation in the extreme W – are the Crim Rocks (2m0) and others near them lying about 1½ miles N of the Bishop Rock. Sailing into these islands in thick weather is extremely dangerous, and the greatest caution is needed when the distant leading marks cannot be positively identified. If in doubt, lie off. The approach to St Mary's Road from the E, which is recommended locally, is by way of St Mary's Sound which is clearly marked. Alternatively approach can be made in suitable weather to Crow Sound from the SE provided the wind is offshore, the bar is not crossed and one anchors to the E of the Hats buoy. At night also, if seeking a lee on the E side of the islands, it may assist to note that Peninnis light becomes obscured on a bearing of about 231°. However, navigation at night is not recommended in the absence of local knowledge.

Approach Channels from the East
Crow Sound (Transit A) The flood tide flows into here, thus the unlit Hats buoy (YB S-cardinal) is left close to starboard, after which Transit A is left to put the rock of Innisidgen Island (7m high), which dries 0m6, clear to port. The Crow Bar Sands, formerly 0m9, have moved and increased. From the Hats buoy steer 289° heading for Green Island, a rock (4m) off the nearest (SE) corner of Tresco. With Bar Point (the northernmost point on St Mary's Island) abeam, course should be altered to 250°, so as to leave the R Bn marking Crow Rocks one cable clear to port. At this point it is safe to alter to port to SW and the deep waters of St Mary's Road. Entry should not be attempted at Springs without ample tide; the best water will be found where sand and weed meet, which can usually be spotted in the clear water.

St Mary's Sound (Transit B) Approach from the SE to avoid Gilston (dries 3m9). The recommended leading marks for this Transit are often difficult to pick up, but there is deep water close to the south of Peninnis Head, with its W pepperpot

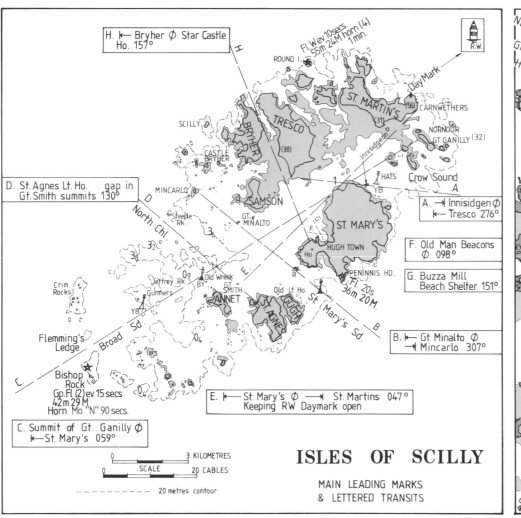

H. ← Bryher ∅ Star Castle
    Ho. 157°

Fl.W.ev.10secs.
55m 24M horn (4)
1 min.

ROUND I.

DayMark
R.W.

SCILLY

TRESCO
(38)

ST. MARTIN'S

CARNWETHERS

(56)

(31)

CASTLE
BRYHER

BRYHER

Innisidgen

NORNOUR
GT.GANILLY (32)

Crow Sound
A

D. St Agnes Lt. Ho.   gap in
   Gt. Smith summits 130°

MINCARLO

SAMSON

HATS
YB

A. → Innisidgen ∅
   ← Tresco 276°

North Chl.

Steeple
Rk.

GT.
MINALTO

ST. MARY'S

F. Old Man Beacons
   ∅ 098°

3²

3⁸

Ho.

HUGH TOWN

G. Buzza Mill
   Beach Shelter 151°

Crim
Rocks

0⁹

Old Wreck
BY

Jeffrey Rk.
Gunners

GT.
SMITH

ANNET

Old Lt. Ho.

R

PENINNIS HD.

Fl. 20s
36m 20M.

St.
Mary's Sd.
B

B. ← Gt. Minalto ∅
   → Mincarlo 307°

YB

ST.
AGNES

0⁴

Flemming's
Ledge

Sd.

Broad

Bishop
Rock
Gp.Fl.(2)ev.15 secs
42m 29M
Horn Mo."N" 90 secs.

E. ← St. Mary's ∅   → St. Martins 047°
   Keeping RW Daymark open.

C. Summit of Gt. Ganilly ∅
   ← St. Mary's 059°

0   3 KILOMETRES

SCALE

0   20 CABLES

— — — — — 20 metres contour

ISLES OF SCILLY

MAIN LEADING MARKS
& LETTERED TRANSITS

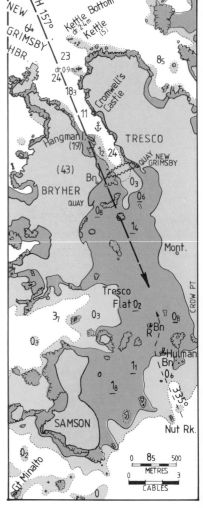

NEW   H 157°
GRIMSBY 64

Kettle Bottom
dr 2·4m

Kettle
(5)

23

24

dr 0·9m

18³

11

Hangman I.
(19)

Cromwell's
Castle

TRESCO

8⁵

HBR

1²·2⁴

QUAY NEW
GRIMSBY

Bn

0³

(43)

BRYHER

0⁶

QUAY

0⁸

1⁴

Mont.

Tresco
Flat 0²

3⁷

0³

0⁸

R Bn

0³

1¹

Hulman
Bn

0⁶

SAMSON

1⁸

CROW PT

335°

Gt. Minalto

0²

Nut Rk.

0   8⁵   500
        METRES
0   3
     CABLES

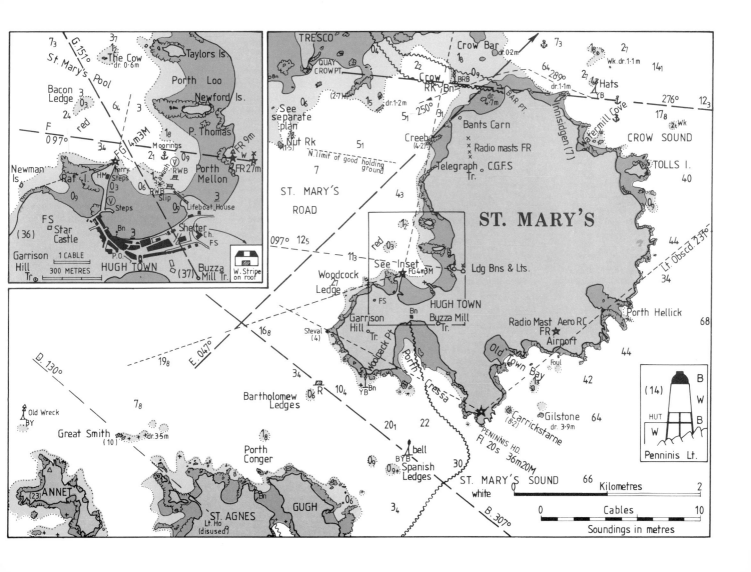

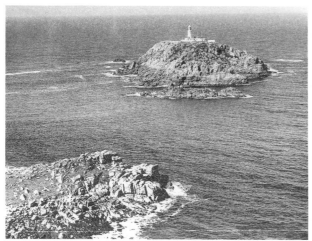

58.1 *Round Island lighthouse (white 19m high, 55m above sea-level) and radio beacon mark the northern extremity of the Scillies.*

lighthouse on a B trellised base (Fl 20s. 36m 20M). The BYB E-cardinal bell buoy marking Spanish Ledges should be left to port, whence the transit course of 307° will leave the R can Bartholomew Ledges buoy close to port. However care should be taken S of Garrison Hill not to get too close to the YB Woolpack Bn, as there is a 0m7 patch ½ cable west of it. Leaving the Bartholomew buoy to port, swing slowly round to the NNE. Deep-draught yachts may want to take Transit E clearing Woodcock Ledge with 2m7 over it.

Approach Channels from the West

Broad Sound (Transit C) leaving Bishop Rock Lt Ho to starboard. The leading marks are over 7 miles away and may not

be identifiable. However, the channel is buoyed starting with the YB south cardinal Gunner buoy, which is left to port. Next make for the N-cardinal Old Wreck BY buoy on course 060°, leaving it to starboard, taking care to keep clear to the SE of the Jeffrey Rock (0m9). The leading marks should now be picked up; they will take the yacht clear to the middle of St Mary's Road.

North Channel (Transit D) A cross-tide may be experienced in the channel, but the leading marks are good in reasonable visibility. The main danger is Steeple Rock (0m4) which is over 6 cables SW of Mincarlo and is left less than 2 cables on the port hand when on the transit of 130°. Stay on it until picking up the Broad Sound Transit C, when course should be altered to 059° into St Mary's Road.

Entrance to St Mary's Pool and Harbour Once in St Mary's Road, most yachts will wish to bring up in the pool. The only danger is the Bacon Ledge (0m3) or Pool Ledge. The former is flanked on the NE by the Cow, which dries 0m6. The most commonly used entry in Transit F on course 097° which brings into line two W Bns N of Porth Mellon, with a triangular topmark on the front one and a cross on the higher rear one, each with an FR Lt. Transit G is from the NW on course 151° between the Cow and Bacon Ledge. It is straightforward, bringing the squat Buzza Mill Tr on the rising ground behind Hugh Town into line with a small shelter on the esplanade, with a W roof and W Vert stripes on either end of its front elevation.

The limit of the anchorage for yachts is roughly a line from the outer quay steps to Newford Island. Yachts should anchor to the SE of this line, keeping clear of the launching area for the lifeboat and leaving plenty of room for the ferry *Scillonian* to turn through 360° after slipping.

An Alternative Anchorage If a blow from the SW is imminent, larger yachts can anchor in Crow Sound ESE of the Hats buoy off Watermill Bay in the NE of St Mary's Island.

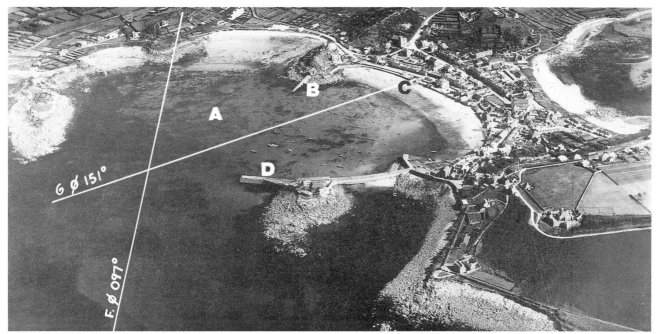

G ∅ 151°

F. ∅ 097°

58.2 *(A) Anchorage for yachts (B) Lifeboat station (C) Hut on the beach which is front leading mark for Transit G (D) Ferry pier where yachts can lie alongside during the ferry's absence, with Harbour Office*

Facilities Although the smaller inhabited islands have little village stores, Hugh Town on St Mary's offers every facility to be found on the mainland, such as a PO, chemist, hospital, provision stores, banks, hotels and bistros. Water and fuel are obtainable on the quay. There are chandlers and boat repairers. Customs are on the quay. Frequent daily helicopter service to Penzance, with connecting bus services from downtown. Ferries leave every afternoon in the summer for Penzance. The HM listens out on Ch 16 or 14; tel. 0720–22768. Yacht club: Isle of Scilly YC.

New Grimsby Harbour – Tresco See Admiralty Chart. This island is famous for its tropical gardens and collection of

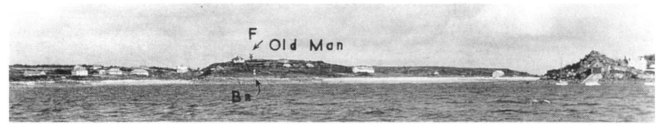

58.3 *Transit F – beacon and The Old Man on skyline*

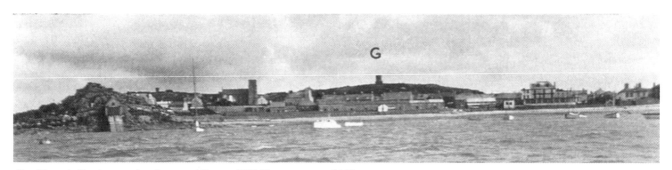

58.4 *Transit G – hut on the shore and Buzza Mill Tower on top of hill*

ships' figureheads. Yachts like to anchor in the passage between the island and Bryher. The entrance from the NW should only be attempted for the first time in favourable weather with a leading wind or under power. Tides up to 2 knots may be experienced. Keep on Transit H and give particular attention to the Kettle and Kettle Bottom Ledges which dry little over a cable to the NE at the entrance, and also to a drying rock which

is inside the entrance but scarcely ½ cable to the NE. There is a deep anchorage in 11m between Cromwell's Castle and Hangman Isle; after this the bottom shoals to 2m4 and then down to 0m3 in the channel opposite the quay at New Grimsby on Tresco, where a dinghy may be left in safety while one is exploring the famous tropical gardens at the S end or the luxurious hotel on the other side of the island at Old Grimsby.

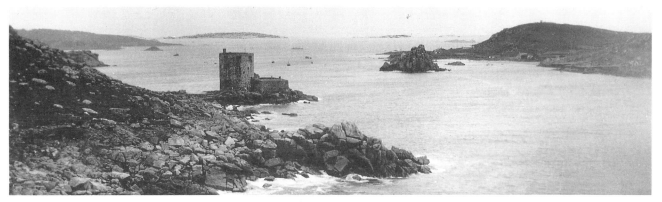

58.5 *Approach H from NNW to Grimsby Harbour. Cromwell's Castle on Tresco Island, with Bryher and Hangman's Island on right and St Mary's in the distance*

Note that a cable, marked by Bns on either side, crosses the channel just NW of the quay. There is an inn and a small shop close to New Grimsby quay.

The passage from St Mary's to New Grimsby looks more formidable than it is. Leave to port the unmarked Nut Rock (2) and the B Hulman Bn close to starboard. Raggs Bn to port, Merrick Island close to port and thence straight to the anchorage. A useful transit between Hulman Bn and Merrick Island is to keep the latter in line with Hangman Isle, then leaving it close to port proceed as before to the anchorage. Tresco Flats dry out between Hulman Bn and the anchorage but these can be crossed by vessels up to 3m draught at HW if precisely on course. On the first occasion a stranger might be wise to treat the flat as drying 1m4. Alternatively, make a reconnaissance by dinghy or in one of the tripper boats which ply between the islands – then consult Norm's book.

Weather BBC shipping forecast area: Sole (Plymouth, Fastnet, Lundy).
Marinecall: 0898–500 458.
Land's End Rdo: VHF Ch 27 or 88 0803 and 2003.

List of Admiralty Chart Agents

***Agents holding comprehensive stocks of corrected Admiralty charts (tel. nos listed).
Most sell Imray and Stanford charts as well – as do all chandleries, especially those in marinas**

United Kingdom

Aberdeen
  *Kelvin Hughes, 21 Regent Quay,
  AB1 2AH, (0224–580823).
  *Thomas Gunn, 62 Marischal Street,
  AB1 2AL, (0224–595045)

Aberdovey
  Dovey Marine, Copperhill Street,
  LL35 0EW

Abersoch
  Abersoch Boatyard Ltd,
  The Saltings, LL53 7AR

Alderney
  Mainbrayce Ltd, Inner Harbour,
  Braye

Aultbea
  Bridgend Stores, Ross and Cromarty,
  IV22 2JA

Avonmouth
  *W F Price & Co Ltd, 24 Gloucester
  Road, BS11 9AD, (0272–823888)

Axminster
  Axminster Chandlery (Leisure) Ltd,
  McNeil House, George Street.

Bangor, North Wales
  A M Dickie & Sons, 36 Garth Road,
  LL57 2SE

Barmouth
  The Seafarer, Church Street,
  LL42 1EH

Belfast
  James Tedford & Co Ltd,
  5 & 9 Donegal Quay, BT1 3EF

Birmingham
  Hollywood Marine Ltd, 15 Highfield
  Road, Hall Green, B28 03L

Boston
  Boston Marina, 5/7 Witham Bank,
  PE21 9JU

Brightlingsea
  L H Morgan & Sons (Marine) Ltd,
  The Boat Centre, 32–42 Waterside,
  CO7 0AY

Brighton
  Russell Simpson Marine Ltd,
  Brighton Marina

Brixham
  Brixham Yacht Supplies, 72 Middle
  Street, TQ5 8EJ

Bromley
  Champion (Bromley Boats) Ltd,
  109–123 Southlands Road, BR2 9QX

Burghead
  Burghead Boat Centre, Burghead
  Harbour, IV30 2VA

Burnham-on-Crouch
  Kelvin Aqua Ltd, The Quay,
  CM0 8AT

Cardiff
  T J Williams & Sons Ltd,
  15/17 Harrowby Street, CF1 6HA
  Blair's Nautical Supplies Ltd,
  28 James Street Docks, CF1 6EX

Chatham
  Gransden Marine, Pier Chambers,
  Medway Street, ME4 4HB

Chichester
  Yacht & Sports Gear, 13 The Hornet
  and the Yacht Basin, PO19 4JL

Christchurch
Rossiter Yacht Builders Ltd, Bridge Street, BH23 1DZ

Cowes
Pascall, Atkey & Son Ltd, 29 High Street, PO31 7RX

Crinan, Argyll
Crinan Boats Ltd, PA31 8SP

Dale, Dyfed
Dale Sailing Co Ltd, SA62 3RB

Dartmouth
The Bosun's Locker, 24 Lower Street, TQ5 9AN

Douglas, Isle of Man
Manx Marine Ltd, 35 North Quay

Dover
Dover Marine Supplies, 158/160 Snargate Street, CT17 9BZ

Dundee
Sea & Shore Marine Supplies, Fish Dock Road, DD1 3LZ

Edinburgh
Chattan Shipping Services Ltd, 5 Canon Mills, EH3 5HA

Emsworth
Castlemain (Marine) Ltd, Emsworth Yacht Harbour, Thorney Road, PO10 8BP

Exeter
Elands, 22 Bedford Street, EX1 1LE

Exmouth
Peter Dixon Chandlery, The Pier, EX8 1DU

Falmouth
*Marine Instruments, Upton Slip, Church Street, TR11 3PS, (0326–312414)

Felixstowe
Small Craft Deliveries Ltd, 34 Orwell Road, IP11 7DB

Fleetwood
The Fleetwood Trawlers Supply Co Ltd, 240/244 Dock Street, FY7 6NU

Fowey
Troy Chandlery, 10 Lostwithiel Street, PL23 1BD

Glasgow
*Kelvin Hughes, 375 West George Street, G2 4LR, (041221–5452)
Christie & Wilson, 70B Dobbie's Lane, G4 0BN

Gloucester
Bellows & Bown, 7 Commercial Road, GL1 1NW

Goodwick, Dyfed
Goodwick Marine Services, 1 Wern Road, Goodwick

Gosport
Hardway Marine, 95–99 Priory Road, Hardway, PO12 4LQ

Great Yarmouth
Gorleston Marine Ltd, Beach Pavilion Road, Gorleston on Sea, NR31 6BY

Grimsby
*Grahams Chart Agency Ltd, Corporation Road, Alexandra Dock, DN31 1VE, (0472–46673)

Guernsey
*Boatworks Plus Ltd, Castle Embankment, St Peter Port, (0481–26071)

Navigation & Marine Supplies, North Plantation, St Peter Port

Holyhead
Holyhead Chandlery, Newry Beach, LL65 1EU

Hull
*B Cooke & Son Ltd, Kingston Observatory, 58/59 Market Place, HU1 1RH, (0482–223454)

Instow
F Johns & Son, Harbourside, The Quay, EX39 4RN

Inverness
Caley Marine and Chandlery, Canal Road, Muirtown, IV3 6NF

Ipswich
Fox's Marina Ipswich Ltd,
The Strand, Wherstead, IP2 8NL

Jersey
South Pier Shipyard, St Helier

Lerwick
Hay & Co (Lerwick) Ltd, 106A
Commercial Street, ZE1 0JD

Liverpool
*Dubois Phillips & McCallum Ltd,
Oriel Chambers, Covent Garden,
L2 8UD, (051-2362776)

J Sewill Ltd, 36 Exchange Street
East, L2 3PT

London
*Kelvin Hughes, 145 Minories,
EC3N 1NH, (071-709 9076)
Capt O M Watts Ltd, 45 Albemarle
Street, W1X 4BJ
London Yacht Centre, 13 Artillery
Lane, E1 7LP
*Brown & Perring Ltd, Redwing
House, 36/44 Tabernacle Street,
EC2A 4DT, (071-253 4517)
Thomas Foulkes, Samson Road,
Leytonstone, E11 3HB
Stanfords International Map Centre,
12/14 Long Acre, WC2E 9LP
Telesonic Marine Ltd, 60-62
Brunswick Centre, Marchmont
Street, London WC1

Lowestoft
*Charity & Taylor (Electronic
Services) Ltd, 4 Battery Green Road,
NR32 1DE, (0502-573943)

Lymington
Nick Cox Yacht Chandler Ltd, Kings
Saltern Road, SO4 9QD

Maldon
Dan Webb & Feesey, North Street,
CM9 7HN

Mallaig
Johnson Brothers, PH41 4QD

Manchester
International Marine, Unit 20-21
Waterway, Enterprise Park, Trafford
Wharf Road, M17 1EY

Middlesborough
Eccles Marine Co Ltd, Saltwater
House, Longlands Road, TS4 2JR

Milford Haven
Westfield Chandlery, Brunel Quay,
Neyland, SA73 1NX

Newhaven
Cantell & Sons Ltd, The Old
Shipyard, Robinson Road, BN9 9BY

North Shields
*John Lilley & Gillie Ltd, Clive
Street, NE29 6LD, (091-2583519)

Nottingham
Starboard, 362 Carlton Hill, NG4 1JB

Oban
Nancy Black, 24/25 Argyll Square,
PA34 4AT

Paignton
Harbour Sports, The Harbour,
TQ4 6DT

Pembroke Dock
Kelpie Boat Services Ltd, Hobbs
Point, SA72 6TR

Plymouth
*A E Monsen, Vauxhall Quay,
PL4 0DT, (0752-665384)

*The Sea Chest Nautical Bookshop,
Queen Anne's Battery Marina,
PL4 0LP (0752-222012)

Poole
H Pipler & Son Ltd, The Quay,
BH15 1HF

Porthmadog
Glaslyn Marine Supplies Ltd,
3 Oakley Wharf, The Harbour,
LL49 9AY

Portsmouth
Gieves & Hawkes Ltd, 21 The Hard,
PO1 3DY

Preston
  Shipsides Marine Ltd, 5 New Hall Lane, PR1 5ND

Pwllheli
  William Partingdon Marine Ltd, The Harbour, LL53 5AY

Ramsgate
  The Bo'sun's Locker, Military Road, CT11 8LN

Rye
  Sea Cruisers Ltd, Winchelsea Road, TN31 7EL

St Leonards on Sea
  Sussex Marine, 48 Marina, TN38 0BE

St Mary's, Isles of Scilly
  Armoral Studio, Garrison Lane, Strand

Salcombe
  Salcombe Chandlers Ltd, 19 Fore Street, TQ8 8BU

Saltash
  Saltash Marine, 2 Regal Court, PL12 6JY

Sheerness
  William Hurst Ltd, 19 West Street, Bluetown, ME12 1SP

Shoreham Harbour
  A O Muggeridge Ltd, 141/143 The Gardens, Southwick, BN4 4DP

Southampton
  *Kelvin Hughes, 19–23 Canute Road, SO1 1FJ, (0703–631286)

Southend-on-Sea
  Shoreline (Yachtsmen) Ltd, 36 Eastern Esplanade, SS1 2ES

Stornoway, Isle of Lewis
  Duncan MacIver Ltd, 7 Maritime Buildings, PA87 2XU

St Ives, Cambs
  Imray Laurie, Norie & Wilson Ltd, Wych House, The Broadway, PE17 4BT

Swansea
  *Cambrian Small Boats & Chandlery & Co Ltd, 14 Cambrian Place, South Dock, SA1 1RG, (0792–467263)

Tarbert
  W B Leitch & Son, Garvel Road, PA29 6TR

Tobermory, Isle of Mull
  Seafare, Portmore Place, PA75 6NU

Topsham
  The Foc'sle, 32 Fore Street, EX3 0HD

Ullapool
  Ullasport, West Argyle Street, IV26 2TY

Upton on Severn
  Upton Marina Chandlery, East Waterside, WR8 0P8

Warsash
  Warsash Nautical Bookshop, 31 Newtown Road, SO3 6FY

Wells-Next-The-Sea
  Standard House (Chandlery) Ltd, Standard House, East Quay, NR23 1JY

West Mersea
  The Mersea Chandlers, 110 Coast Road, CO5 8NB

Weymouth
  W L Bussell, 11 Nothe Parade, DT4 8TX

Whitby
  M R Coates (Marine), The Boatyard, Esk Terrace, YO21 1EU

Whitstable
  The Dinghy Store, Sea Wall, CT5 1BX

Woodbridge
  *Small Craft Deliveries Ltd, 12 Quay Street, IP12 1BX, (03943–2600)

Republic of Ireland

Cork
Union Chandlery Ltd, Andersons
Quay

Dublin 2
*Windmill Leisure & Marine Ltd,
3 Windmill Lane, Sir John
Rogerson's Quay, (77 2008)

Galway
Galway Maritime Services,
New Docks

France

Harfleur 76700
(near Le Havre)
*Nautic Service SARL, Zac de
Rogerville Oudalle, (35.51.75.30)

Paris 75006
Librairie Maritime et d'Outre-Mer,
17 Rue Jacob, 6e
Librairie Nautique et Des Voyages,
6 Rue de Mézières, 6e

Paris 75009
L'Astrolabe, La Librairie Du
Voyager, 46 Rue De Provence, 9e